Prais

M000282150

'Like Janey herself, Happy Healthy Sober *is fabulously upbeat, wise and fun. I defy you to read this book and not want to be a part of Janey's sober gang.'*
Clare Pooley, author of *The Sober Diaries*

'In Happy Healthy Sober, *Janey provides a personal, unique and most importantly fun guide to having a fabulous alcohol-free life. She gives you the keys to making sobriety and a healthy lifestyle cool, memorable and tremendously appealing. It is a breath of fresh air.'*
Dr Gemma Newman

'A fabulous book from Janey Lee Grace and the perfect book for 2021.'
Jo Wood, author and TV personality
(Founder of Jo Wood's Organics)

'A truly enlightening read, you'll never look back.'
Jason Vale, author, speaker, pro-juicer

'This book has been written just at the right time and could be the difference between desire for change and actually finding the discipline to change.'
Carrie Grant MBE

'Janey really hits the mark with Healthy Happy Sober, *it's not just a book about quitting drinking, but about getting every ounce of joy and pleasure from life.'*
William Porter, author of *Alcohol Explained*

'As I know from experience. when you are changing your drinking hab-its it is not just one thing that works. So Janey's book is brilliant at bringing together experts with all sorts of ideas about how you can create and sustain change for the long term. Enjoy!'
Laura Willoughby MBE

'A helpful, knowledgeable book for anyone looking to discover that sobriety truly does rock.'
Annie Grace, author of *This Naked Mind: Control Alcohol, Find Freedom, Discover Happiness & Change Your Life*

'This book is about how to feel buzzed without booze. Janey knows a thing or two about ditching the booze. Her new book throws a new light on this important subject. Janey gives so many useful ideas and life hacks to help embracing living alcohol-free for those who are struggling in this area.

This is a great read for people who want to manage their relationship with alcohol and get some solid support in the process. Easy to read, full of great material. Highly recommended.'
Susie Pearl, author and podcaster on happiness, wellness and creativity

'In our alcohol-based culture, Janey Lee Grace has provided the other badly needed side of the story that has been conspicuous by its absence. And she's done it without the po-faced earnest suffering tone one would expect from a book promoting not being tipsy and even not drinking at all.'
Dr Aric Sigman

'A book that the future you will thank you for reading. Happy Healthy Sober is a fantastic resource for an alcohol-free life, packed with resources to support your mind, heart, body and soul.'
Andy Coley, International NLP Trainer – Beyond NLP

'Want to be happy, healthy and sober? Janey Lee Grace has the answers to set you on a path to a new and better way of living. But more than that, her well earned life wisdom is an elixir of transformational tools to create a new, better and wiser you. Guaranteed after you read this book, your glass will never be half empty again.'
Kate Delamere, writer, editor and journalist

HAPPY HEALTHY SOBER

Ditch the booze and take control of your life

Janey Lee Grace

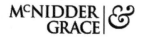

MᶜNIDDER | & GRACE

To my beloved hubby Simon and our gorgeous kids,
Sonny, Buddy, Rocky and Lulu

Published by McNidder & Grace
21 Bridge Street
Carmarthen
SA31 3JS
Wales, UK

www.mcnidderandgrace.com
First published in 2021
Reprinted 2021
© Janey Lee Grace

Janey Lee Grace has asserted her right to be identified as the author of this work in accordance with the Copyright, Designs and Patents Act 1988.

The information given in this book is intended for general purposes only. It is not intended as and should not be relied upon as medical advice; always consult a medical practitioner. Any use of information in this book is at the reader's discretion and risk. Neither the author nor the publisher can be held responsible for any loss, claim or damage arising out of the use, misuse, of the suggestions made, the failure to take medical advice or for any material from third party contributors.

Every effort has been made to obtain necessary permission with reference to copyright material. The publisher apologises if, inadvertently, any sources remain unacknowledged and will be glad to make the necessary arrangements at the earliest opportunity.

A catalogue record for this work is available from the British Library.

ISBN: 9780857162120
Ebook: 9780857162137

Designed by JS Typesetting Ltd
Cover design: Lara Peralta

Printed and bound in the United Kingdom by Short Run Press Ltd, Exeter, UK

CONTENTS

Foreword   ix

Introduction   1

PART 1

Chapter 1   The eternal search for peace and happiness   5
Chapter 2   A high bottomed gal, and at least 50 shades
of grey   11
Chapter 3   I gave up for Dry January and never went back   15
Chapter 4   Get the buzz without the booze   23
Chapter 5   Preparing to ditch the drink   29
Chapter 6   Breaking the habit. The first 7 days   41
Chapter 7   The next 30 days!   45
Chapter 8   Checking in   55
Chapter 9   Self-care, sleep, relaxation, exercise   57
Chapter 10   Getting social – how to deal with relationships
and the social scene   61
Chapter 11   Sober drinking   67
Chapter 12   Setting goals. Journaling and vision boards   71

PART 2

Chapter 13   Stages of Change   77
Chapter 14   Sober Healthy Living   81
Chapter 15   The Sober Mind   115
Chapter 16   The Sober Heart   133
Chapter 17   The Sober Body   147
Chapter 18   The Sober Soul   169
Chapter 19   The Sober Lifestyle   179

Afterword   Be a rocking sober badass!   197

Bibliography and recommended reading   201

Contributors   205

Recommended resources   207

Acknowledgements   212

About the author   213

FOREWORD

I had my last drink in April 2012. Next year I will have been sober for 9 years. Apart from my children it is the thing that makes me most proud. Not only for myself but for the people who love me.

I know we are all experiencing difficult times in so many ways and the temptation to drink is greater than ever. But honestly, if consuming alcohol is no longer a fun way to spend time with friends and have a laugh, if it's hurting your relationships with the people you love, if you are rowing with your partner and neither of you can remember, then you may have a problem. If your anger is directed at those who point out that you have a problem… then you probably do. It is never too late to stop. Trust me, you don't stop being funny, you probably weren't funny a lot of the time anyway, you just thought you were! You don't lose confidence, you gain it as you reclaim your self-esteem. Nights out are still fun, you will probably leave early (driving) and get home in time for a cuppa and a crumpet and 3 hours to watch crap telly before bed.

I'm not the drink police, believe me, but increasingly I have people asking me about getting sober. My advice – it's hard, but it's so worth it.

I would rather go through life sober and believing I am an alcoholic than go through life drunk and believing I'm not.

There are plenty of resources and communities out there to help you. And Janey's *Happy Healthy Sober* book will certainly help you to ditch the booze and take more control of your life. Janey focuses on the huge benefits of sobriety and how this will improve your health and wellbeing. With Janey's experience, and with contributions from leading experts, all that is needed to succeed is the commitment from you.

Go on, do it. I know you can. I promise you won't look back.

Denise Welch 2021

INTRODUCTION

Are you thinking of ditching the booze?

Have you often asked yourself the question: Would my life be better physically and emotionally without alcohol?

If the answer is 'Hell, yes!' or even…'I think it could be', make a decision to ditch the booze – even if only for a short period of time.

Let me convince you why you should quit the booze even for a bit.

> *Ya think that the whiskey tastes good? Try a big cup of sobriety – now that is the good stuff!*
>
> Steven Tyler

Sobriety rocks!

Being alcohol-free is without doubt the new cool.

Forget any perceptions you may have of the sad ex drinker who 'can't ever have a drink'. You *can* have a drink; not having one is *your choice*.

This is a book about how so very cool it is to be alcohol-free. I will share my story about giving up, and help you in detail through the all-important first week, first month and beyond. You will find it hard sometimes, you will question everything, and you will wonder what you have started as you shift and settle into the 'new you'.

I will encourage you to try new types of non-alcoholic drinks. I will help you find your purpose and enjoy getting fit and healthy again. I will introduce you to some awesome sober heroes who share their tips for sobriety. And if you've been searching for that 'missing piece', I hope to show you it may well be the very thing that's got you in denial. If reading this is giving you a slightly uncomfortable feeling, stay with me for the ride; I promise you it will be worth it.

Part One

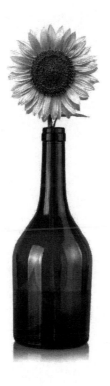

Chapter 1
THE ETERNAL SEARCH FOR PEACE AND HAPPINESS

I'm someone known for her recommendations for all things health and wellbeing, so there isn't much in the health, wellness and spirituality arena that I haven't sampled. In 2006, with my first book, *Imperfectly Natural Woman*, I was a little ahead of my time. I was writing about organic, extra virgin coconut oil as a fabulous hair conditioner and moisturiser long before celebs were using it liberally and teaching us oil pulling techniques for whiter teeth. I was a devotee of green juices and smoothies long before Kale and Turmeric had their own publicist. And while not heralding myself as especially green, I sure knew about sustainability and ethical living. I was passionate about mindset and spirituality too, and later wrote *Look Great Naturally... Without Ditching the Lipstick* published by Hay House, known for their motivational books.

All this has required me to keep ahead of the curve. To be across not only the latest organic skincare, superfoods and supplement trends, but also to find out what treatments and therapies work, and to explore the latest coaching models and meditation techniques in the quest for peace, happiness, and optimum health and wellbeing.

I'm queen of it *all*! I live and breathe it, and I wish I could say I only went along to the next therapist, or accepted a session with the latest NLP coach, in order to write reviews for my blog. The real truth, though, is that I continued to seek out these opportunities because I wanted to see if anyone or anything could fix me.

Over the 12 years I have been practising holistic living, I have been on at least 10 detox retreats and attended workshops courses and classes on everything from meditation to NLP to kindness and happiness. I have been constantly striving to be a better version of myself, to find the peace that always eluded me. I suffered from anxiety, and almost always felt fearful. I blamed my childhood. My parents were not unloving; they just didn't seem available to me, suffering themselves from mental illness and a kind of fear of life. I rarely felt secure, and as so often happens to women who haven't had a close relationship with their father, I looked for a father figure, which meant that I stayed in a verbally abusive relationship far longer than I should have done. Prior to writing my first wellbeing book I met my husband, the father of my four children, and I found security and true love – but still there was something missing. Peace and happiness and the ability to have fun.

I have done yoga for years, I have tried meditation and taken relaxation classes, I've watched copious amounts of TEDx Talks, attended Hay House conferences and consumed vast quantities of media from the likes of Wayne Dyer and Deepak Chopra. Even before working with Hay House (where an author perk is fabulous free books!), I had amassed the most massive 'shelf help' library – you know what I mean; they all stay on the shelf, dipped into but rarely helping to effect change.

I have tried shamanic healing, transformational hypnotherapy, sessions with an angel practitioner, EFT (Emotional Freedom Techniques), TFT (Thought Field Therapy), soul coaching, tarot reading, energy healing, aura cleansing. I've even worked with a healer who could see my 'Akashic records' – my former lives and the 'contracts' that needed to break in order for me to be fully present and prosper in this life.

For mind and bodywork I have had aromatherapy, crystal therapy, reiki healing, regular progressive kinesiology sessions (it's magical; by muscle testing and a fair amount of intuition the therapist can 'talk' to your body and emotions and know what's needed – sounds bonkers, doesn't it). I've had Bowen technique, chiropractic, myofascial release, Rolfing, Amatsu – I could go on…

I hired a Feng Shui expert to dowse and 'space clear' my home.

I ensured that there was good chi in my health area, and energy flowing to my wealth corner. I fitted grounding devices, had tests for excessive electromagnetic frequencies and installed harmonisers to deflect the radiation from Wi-Fi and computers et al. I festooned my home with the right house plants (peace lilies are great for removing formaldehyde to a range of 9 metres/30 feet, and cacti are great to have by your computer).

I've been to nutritionists, had a personalised health plan and a DNA test (which seemed to say that one or two alcoholic drinks are good for my genetic profile...WTF?), and I have tried just about every supplement, mineral, vitamin and tonic there is in order to find my optimum state of health. If it weren't for the fact that I was doing a lot of this as a journalist and in the name of research, you'd call me one of the seriously worried well.

I was always searching, seeking, praying, and hoping for answers. In the last couple of years before I stopped drinking, I knew something was really wrong: I was often anxious, sleeping badly and waking up at 3 a.m., full of self-loathing, my heart beating fast, as I prayed to someone, anyone who could take this curse away. I regularly planned alcohol-free days, and then failed miserably as soon as the clock hit 6 p.m., the 'appropriate' time to have the first drink.

I was starting to feel antsy and fearful, achieving less, feeling more anxious and being irritable a lot of the time. I was overweight, had digestive problems and looked a bit bloated. Every time I saw a new healer or tried a new treatment, I had high hopes that this time I'd be fixed, made whole. I don't know what magic button I expected would be pressed, but it sure as hell never was.

On some of my treatment sessions, the nutritionist, therapist, or healer would ask about my diet and alcohol consumption. Of course, I lied about the amount I drank – who doesn't? And they'd nod and say that seems fine, a couple of glasses of wine won't hurt. Even the GP told me I had nothing to worry about. In the last couple of years, I started tentatively to speak out. At the end of our session the therapist would say: 'Is there anything else you'd like to look at? Is there anything you'd like me to ask the angels/spirit guides on your behalf?' I'd admit with shame that I thought I might be drinking too much, that I had a voice in my head which seemed to force me to go back for a second and third glass of wine, and that I couldn't seem to make it go away.

I was advised to go back in my mind to my childhood and look at what might be making me feel out of control. I was told I might have attracted a demonic entity which was making me drink too much (there's a reason certain drinks are called spirits apparently!) and I was advised to carry crystals to protect myself. In case you aren't well versed in all this woo-woo, an entity is a being that has been created from negativity, and which brings chaos and mischief. I sure did have that going on!

I was constantly searching, always in the pursuit of the answer. I always wanted more – more happiness, more contentment, more love, more fun and more peace. I knew, because I had met Louise Hay and read most of her work, the importance of loving myself, and I wrote many a blog post on self-esteem. But I didn't love myself very much at all. In fact, when I dragged my exhausted ass out of bed in the morning, cautiously at first as I tried to ascertain whether the room was spinning or not, I actually disliked myself – a lot. None of this sat well with the label I wore: 'holistic living expert'. It didn't feel very authentic; I wondered when I'd be found out.

I carried on doing everything I could to find a way to love myself, everything other than looking, really looking at my relationship with alcohol – and no one else, even the most enlightened of light workers, shone a light on it either.

Not once, did anyone ever talk to me, *really* talk to me about the fact that alcohol is a poison, and that if like me and millions of others, you can't moderate that poison, it will make you anxious and fearful and you won't feel whole ... and will be on the slippery slope down to hell. In fairness I didn't identify and present myself to any of these fixers as having an issue with alcohol; I was always complaining about less specific issues. I couldn't possibly come out and book a session with anyone to discuss the very real problem of drinking too much. It was the elephant in the room. Why didn't I face it? Why didn't they tell me?

Because alcohol is *everywhere!* Because those therapists, coaches and doctors were probably drinking themselves, possibly too much. Because it's ingrained in our society to such an extent that unless you are an actual alcoholic (usually defined in the popular imagination as someone who is completely down and out and in need of or going to Alcoholics Anonymous) then you're 'just fine.'

No one takes into account the shades of grey that make up the reality for so many drinkers. They aren't rock bottom *yet*, but they are lacking energy and feeling stuck, disempowered and fearful.

Do you know what else no one told me?

How freaking fantastic life without alcohol really is. Sobriety rocks!

Chapter 2
A HIGH BOTTOMED GAL, AND AT LEAST 50 SHADES OF GREY

There is a huge rise in the number of people facing up to their issues with alcohol.

Since discovering the 'sober community' – the growing number of people of all ages from all over the globe who are making the decision to remove alcohol from their lives and are finding that life is actually better – I have felt very supported. Even so, I have also come across a lot of words and labels that I dislike.

Let's start with the word *alcoholic*. If you're happy with that moniker for yourself, who am I to bicker? Trouble is, I, and probably a large percentage of my peer group, once thought that there were two types of people: alcoholics, those who have a dysfunctional relationship with alcohol and who are addicts with a lifelong disease; and those who are perfectly fine, and can drink socially without ever descending into that slippery abyss. I now know differently. I know that there are those who are at rock bottom (low bottom drunks), but there are many shades of grey. I now know I am (or was) high bottomed. A phrase I am happy to own. Oh how I wish I actually did have a pert derriere! Sadly, it's going slowly south with the rest of me as I age (gracefully). But I realise now that I was still relatively near the top of that long descent and for that I am eternally grateful.

So no, I don't want to refer to myself as an alcoholic. The reality is that choosing not to drink brings a wonderful freedom. I'll talk later about the reaction of friends, family and work colleagues when it finally dawns on them that you have stopped drinking, but however supportive they are, you don't usually get the round of applause that comes if you've given up smoking.

'*Well done you,*' they cheer, when you finally crack your twenty-a-day habit. '*Congratulations! You overcame the demon nicotine, let's celebrate!*'

We rarely label smokers addicted to nicotine a *nicoholic*; we rally round and pat them on the back. Sadly, it's not the same with alcohol but I would rather identify as being *alcohol-free* or even a *non-alcoholic*.

When we quit drinking, however, the assumption is that we surely must have been sad, sorry, secret, rock-bottom alcoholics.

'*You've stopped drinking? Oh, poor you, did you have a problem? Was it awful for you? How bad did it get?*' Usually quickly followed by '*Well, just have one...that won't hurt, don't be boring.*'

Alcohol is a drug – and a pretty powerful one at that. Stats, which most of us would really rather not look at, show that it's actually more harmful than crack cocaine and heroin. I know we aren't comparing like with like given that alcohol is legal and has been for centuries, but two separate studies have concluded that alcohol is the most dangerous drug in the UK, primarily because of its harm to others, including the wider economy. But it's so integrated into our society that we feel we have to justify ourselves if we don't drink it!

The word *sober* is another word I used to dislike. Have you noticed it's an anagram of *bores*? I was very conscious that I didn't want to appear boring; I was 'good old Janey, the life and soul of the party', for God's sake. '*We love Janey when she's taken a drink, she's hilarious,*' they insisted. Well, you know what, I am still the same person, I can still have fun. In fact, I have come to learn that without the crippling haze of booze I can really enjoy myself, but I won't waste my time anymore on people who really are loathsome or boring, whether they are sober or not. Over time as the 'sober community' has grown in all its glorious technicolour, I'm cool with the label 'sober' – just don't call me boring!

Recovery and *rehabilitation* also have connotations of desperation, an impossible uphill struggle, a long process that can't be made without professional help and with huge shame at its core. 'They tried to make me go to rehab,' sang Amy Winehouse, and it seemed to me that a whole swathe of music lovers patted themselves on the back for not being in that terrible state themselves.

I am going to be talking in this book about *recovery*, despite not being a fan of the word. As I've already indicated, this won't be a drunken memoir, where you will be able to marvel at the horrors of my antics as an old lush. I'll tell you the reality of course, but it's not that grim. I can recommend lots of other Quit Lit – a new phrase I do love, for memoirs from people who have found sobriety; perfect if you do want to revel in the degradation of seemingly high-functioning individuals. But after a whizz through the reasoning for making my decision to stop drinking, I want to focus on the journey to wellness, and the joy of living an alcohol-free life.

I started with Dry January, and never went back to drinking. I credit that to the support network I found, and the sober tools I was able to arm myself with. I've already alluded to the sober community; we are a growing army and will soon be a force to be reckoned with. It wouldn't surprise me if between five and ten years from now, drinking will be the new smoking. Alcohol will finally be outed as the dangerous poison it really is.

If you have been hammering the booze to whatever extent, you will need to prioritise a recovery period. But practise self-care and some of the fabulous health strategies in this book, and you will find yourself within a few months feeling literally like a different person.

Alcohol takes away your energy, dulls your senses and makes you secretive, sluggish, fearful and ashamed. It can damage your health, your relationships and your wallet.

Choosing not to drink makes you feel hopeful, as though things are possible again; it makes you feel proud and powerful, conscious and brave.

This is a time of truth and authenticity, there's no doubt. Millennials are the enlightened ones when it comes to alcohol, it seems; a recent survey found that over 27 per cent of millennials choose to be teetotal. It's the middle-aged who are hammering it, and sadly it's the women who now do more than their fair share of drinking. In my mother's day, Valium may have been doled out indiscriminately, now wine is universally accepted as 'mummy's little helper'. Wine o'clock is the social glue that binds us to friends, neighbours and parenting networks. 'Baby on the hips, wine on the lips' is the mantra. Frazzled mums all around are quaffing the prosecco (their mummy juice) to get them through the exhausting roller coaster of parenting.

All of this comes with a cost, and it's thought that the cost of alcohol use in the UK to the NHS and emergency services is around £4 million.

I don't expect this book to shake any trees for the big guys; I'm not suggesting prohibition or even changing the opening times of pubs. What I would like to do is speak directly to you if you know – whether you have been open about it or whether you have kept it as your own miserable secret for years – that you are drinking too much. Alcohol is controlling you. When once it made you light and joyful, dizzy and witty, now it makes you sad – and scared. The bottle that was once your friend has definitely turned enemy. I want to encourage you to stop drinking and start living. You will feel as though it's impossible, at first, because recovered addicts talk only about how hard it is. But after the initial period, which can be made much easier with support, you will emerge like a butterfly from your cocoon and you will find that life without is so much better. You will find freedom and a joy you didn't think was possible. You will find yourself again.

Chapter 3
I GAVE UP FOR DRY JANUARY AND NEVER WENT BACK

I have already alluded to the fact that I wasn't a rock bottom drunk. I doubt whether anyone noticed I had an issue at all. Sure, I'd quaff down the lion's share of the wine if we went out to dinner with friends; yes, I'd always be the one jumping up to get another round if we had drinks after work. And maybe my local wine bar did consider closing after I stopped going there, such was my nightly spending, and OK, as soon as my teenage boys turned 18 they proudly took their ID cards and bought me wine for my birthday or Christmas. But if you'd asked any of my friends or family, I don't think they would have said they thought I was addicted or that I had any kind of alcohol dependency. I think my husband probably got a bit fed up with me hogging the conversation when I was onto my third glass of wine, but everyone was so loud by then, it didn't seem to matter. I very rarely had so much that I threw up (there was one occasion after a BBC party, but I've almost blocked that from my memory) and I didn't ever drink and drive. (Though I did drive the morning after once and afterwards felt terrified when I realised I could still have been over the limit.) I didn't get maudlin or angry when I was drunk, and I could usually (I think) remember what I had said and done.

I didn't start drinking too early in my teens. I'm grateful for that: I read with some horror Dr Aric Sigman's book *Alcohol Nation*,

15

in which he reveals that children as young as 8 are drinking. I guess I started at around 16 and I didn't particularly like it. Over time, like most students, I taught myself how to like white wine and eventually red wine, but I was never a beer drinker and it was only in the last year before I stopped drinking that I started on the gin and tonics.

At first I was a 'normie', the name we alcohol-free types give to those normal people who can have one drink and who don't drink every day – not because they are frantically forcing themselves to think about something else, but because they don't even think about it. I don't know what changed. When I was touring around the world with bands, the wine and champagne flowed freely, but apart from one awful experience drunk on champagne (never liked it since), and one even more awful experience drunk on sake in Japan (definitely didn't touch it again), I didn't particularly overdo the booze. For the record, I didn't hit the drugs either, though plenty around me did: I was surrounded for years by musos rolling up lines of cocaine and taking cannabis. I can honestly say I was never tempted. I was afraid of drugs (oh, the irony, now I know that alcohol is the most harmful drug of them all!), but I was too scared to lose control, too scared that it would mess with my head. Yet I allowed alcohol to do just that, and while alcohol was a good friend for a good few years – always there when I was feeling a bit down, or when I was feeling good and celebrating – eventually it turned and bit me on the bum.

When my hubby and I bought our first home, the drinking escalated. He is a normie; I think I'm a little jealous of him. He can literally have a glass or two of wine with dinner, even a few too many every now and then at a party, but then he won't think about the booze for days, even weeks. There is no emotional attachment, no voice in his head saying: 'Go on, have another one, it won't hurt.' He can literally nurse one glass of wine throughout a whole dinner party (incredible) and has no concept that some of us just don't seem to have an off switch.

Before the kids came along, you could say we were living the dream. I was working in TV and for Virgin Radio, he was working as a composer and we spent our money on great food and decent wine. Many a bottle of Barolo was consumed in some Italian restaurant in London before my 2 a.m. shift at Virgin, where I sounded fabulously jolly on the air. We threw parties all the time, and always stocked up with copious amounts of alcohol. No one ever needed to bring a bottle; in fact, we discouraged it.

When we moved house after our second child was born, I remember the neighbours looking on quizzically as removal men humped in crate after crate of alcohol to line our lovely wine cellar – a fabulous new addition!

I had the odd drink through all four pregnancies too (seems a bit of a shocker now) and I also didn't stop during breastfeeding, I'd still have the odd glass. In fact, I remember midwives and health visitors recommending I drink Guinness and Coke to boost my breast milk. I hated the taste of Guinness but I took that as all the permission I needed to have the odd tipple of vino.

When my first two boys were young, it was full on: I was presenting radio shows 6 days a week, and doing TV on the seventh day. I was often exhausted and frazzled and started to 'need' a drink as the sun passed over the yard arm. Once we had four children, life was manic, it's fair to say, and I really valued the times I got to feel 'grown-up'. If we had childcare, it felt like a huge treat to be able to go out for a drink. Our local deli had a wine bar, and it became a nightly routine to pop round and get in some me time. Sometimes I would take a magazine and sit there, drinking my large glass of Sauvignon blanc, telling myself I would only have one, but then the bartender would suggest a refill and a voice came from somewhere (moi?) saying: 'Yes please.'

There were times when I started to feel concerned that I was drinking every day. I read about the need for alcohol-free days and tried to plan them. I'd wake up feeling groggy from the night before and decide that this is the day, it's only Tuesday, after all ... but by 6 p.m. something would have kicked off, or we needed to discuss something, hubby would suggest having a quick one – and off we would go.

You might think that weekdays would be best for alcohol-free days. But ... Mondays I did a radio show and it felt really celebratory after a good interview to toast it with a drink; Tuesdays nothing special happened usually, but I did like to relax if I had been at the BBC all day; Wednesdays, well, it was the middle of the week, always worth celebrating; I was often invited to functions or drinks parties on Thursdays; Fridays were our date nights at our favourite restaurant, and of course we shared a bottle of wine (well, actually we didn't, hubby had one small glass and I polished off the rest). And then, well, it was the weekend, so it would be rude not to drink on a Saturday night, whether out with friends or watching *The Voice* with the kids, and Sunday? Well, Sunday means long boozy lunches and a few in the evening while getting ready for the week ahead.

I don't think I ever actually added up how much I drank. I think I'm still in denial. Save to say it must have been pushing five to six bottles of wine a week, and that's not counting the wine I had out in cafés and wine bars. I was rarely drunk, though. That's the thing with big drinkers, they develop a huge tolerance, the body is amazing, it soldiers on, until – well, until it doesn't anymore. I'm incredibly grateful I didn't get to that point.

I didn't think I had too many symptoms. Of course, looking back, I can see that I had lots: I was jittery, bloated, slept really badly, could hardly ever get my contact lenses in, my eyes were often blurry. I felt really quite unfit towards the end of the drinking days, even finding yoga positions that I had been doing for years, too much. I put it all down to getting older. My anxiety was increasing; from moments of sheer panic and terror, I woke often, unable to remember what had scared me. The 3 a.m. wake-ups were the worst: I'd sit up, dry throat and sweating, detesting myself for drinking again.

Sometimes I cried myself back to sleep. I was so upset, disgusted, despairing that something seemingly so simple as just stopping, proved impossible to me once daylight had arrived again. My husband lay beside me, snoring and farting and with absolutely no idea of my turmoil. By 5 p.m. the next evening I was fully sober and ready to start again.

And I couldn't share it with anyone, I was deeply ashamed. Back then, I didn't ever think about giving up forever; that seemed way too forever-ish. Impossible, how could I ever be part of the in-crowd if I was teetotal? How could I enjoy a barbeque on a sunny day without a glass of wine? What would I do at functions?

No, I wasn't interested in abstinence, but I wanted a magic pill to help me take back control of my drinking. I wanted to be like my husband and some of my friends, able to drink one, or none, and this not be an issue.

I quit for a while after reading Jason Vale's book *Kick the Drink ... Easily!* This came directly after a spell at one of Jason's fab juice retreats, so I was feeling wonderfully healthy and 'clean' and it seemed easy just to change my relationship with alcohol. I went on a bit of a raw food trip, and was uber-healthy for a good few months, till some stress crept in and I fancied a glass of wine. Well, I had been without for a couple of months, so I figured that now I could moderate my intake. Wrong. I had one the first night, two the next, and lo and behold I was back on the roller coaster ride – but this time it didn't seem so thrilling and a part of me knew I was falling.

You may be wondering why, if I read that book and changed my mindset, I relapsed and drank again. It's because I hadn't consciously embraced the concept of choosing to be alcohol-free, I hadn't committed, and I certainly didn't put in place any support or tools to get me through it when the wine witch flew back in on her broomstick.

So what changed? I've already said that no one suggested I stop, and I'm unsure what I would have said to them if they had, I would probably have thrown a hissy fit! I spent a lot of time trying to find assurance for my views that drinking is perfectly fine. Oh, how I laughed when Dame Sally Davies claimed that even two drinks a day could mean an increased risk of cancer. Ridiculous, I'd say, it's doing me no harm. In fairness, I did function well. I had masses of energy, was never really ill, and never missed deadlines, but I was starting to feel like two people. There was the Janey who could remember her ambitions and dreams, and then there was the scared Janey who found it easier just to open a bottle of wine and chill out. As is often the case, it was a health scare that got me thinking. I was offered the opportunity to write about thermography and as someone who has never had a mammogram (despite an invite popping through the door on my 50th) I wanted to give it a try. I didn't for one second think my breasts would be anything less than A1, so I got a bit of a shock when the scans showed a potential marker. The optimum number is 1–2 and in one breast I had a marker of 4. The practitioner, a natural doctor, checked for structural changes, said there were none, and suggested it was nothing sinister, but that we would monitor it for six months. Meanwhile, I was to take supplements.

I left feeling very insecure indeed. It wasn't a bad diagnosis as they go – he said lots of women have the same result and six months later it's all good – but I kept on thinking. *What if in six months I go back, and it* is *breast cancer? What then? What will I be saying to myself?* The answer was clear. I would say, *'You should have stopped drinking.'* I just didn't know how to. There never seemed to be the right time.

We had a party a couple of weeks before Christmas and I quaffed back copious amounts of mulled wine and white wine, white wine and finished up with gin and tonic. The next day I went to work (my poor body) and was given a book to read before we came back to work after the Christmas break because we were going to interview the author on 2 January. The book was *The Sober Diaries* by Clare Pooley, based on her blog *Mummy Was a Secret Drinker*.

It was as if the universe was working to wake me up. I knew I had to give healing my potential breast problem my best shot, and as I started to read the book, I had a strange feeling that this was it. This book was going to change my life.

Change my life it did. It seemed to have come at the time I was ready, and I loved the fact that the author insisted life was better without alcohol. I was ready to try.

I had my last drink on 30 December 2017. No one batted an eye when I offered to drive on New Year's Eve to a party. As the designated driver, not drinking was no biggie for me, but I felt a euphoria I hadn't felt in years as I woke up bright and early on New Year's Day. I went out for a long walk to think long and hard about what lay ahead. It was convenient that Dry January was a-rocking. I could work with that, see what happened next.

I didn't tell anyone for the first 30 days. A few people saw me opt for fizzy water and just assumed Dry January, no big deal, and my kids didn't notice. Probably because from the off I armed myself with some non-alcoholic drinks and served them in a wine glass – so it wasn't obvious I wasn't drinking. I liked it that way, I felt really fragile and actually a bit weird for that first month and I definitely couldn't discuss what was going on, it felt too important, too big. I had to keep it close to my heart.

I don't recommend that now. As Johann Hari's famous TED Talk says: 'Connection is the opposite of addiction'. It's hard trying to do it alone. I now encourage you to find your tribe of like-minded people, get the inspiration and support you need.

I'm going to share some of the lessons that might help you navigate the first 30 days.

One of the things holding us back is that we just can't imagine a life without booze, and if we do, we can only imagine it will be worse, we will feel left out, we will be the Cinderella who can't go to the ball. We envisage a dim future; that's it for the fun-loving gal, her party days are over. People tend to focus on what they are giving up rather than what they are gaining.

I hope this book will encourage you that life without the booze is better, infinitely preferable. In fact, it's beautiful, joyous and authentic. You *can* get the buzz without the booze.

Chapter 4
GET THE BUZZ WITHOUT THE BOOZE

So how do you stop drinking and get the buzz without the booze? Let's face it, most of us drink out of habit, and because, well, we like the taste of alcohol (we have become accustomed to it) and we like the feeling it give us. We like the fact that when we have a had a drink it takes the edge off, we can appear more confident, we can let our hair down. So, can you get the buzz without booze? Most of us think we get a buzz from alcohol and this leads to us thinking we need this to feel happy and confident, or relaxed and chilled, or sexy and glamorous, the list goes on. I hope I am going to convince you that it's all an illusion and you absolutely don't need alcohol in your life at all. It's entirely possible to get the buzz without booze. Not only can you survive without drinking alcohol; you can absolutely thrive. These tips will inspire you to live your best life free from the booze.

There are lots of challenges you can work through to help you give up. This is more of a mini course to get you prepared and fully committed to changing your habit of drinking. As with anything in life, the more preparation you do, the more success you're likely to have.

If you're like me, you will have tried reducing or quitting the booze before and ended up going right back to square one! I've learnt that if you lay some foundations, and make some preparations both mentally and physically, you have a much greater chance of success. But I also believe that a focus on how great life is going to be on the other side will give you a better reason for sticking at it. I believe it's not only about ditching the drink, though that's a fabulous start, it's about upscaling your life generally. Often it's only when you stop drinking that you realise there is other stuff you want to do. This is often the time when people become interested in nutrition, fitness and mental wellbeing, or find new hobbies and start new relationships and careers. In other words, they find a purpose.

It's important to stress that I don't know what stage you are at, so if you have already stopped drinking, don't go back to it! The tips, resources and motivation in this section will underpin everything for you, and hopefully you will find new ways to thrive sober. I'd love it if you were able to renew your sense of purpose.

Important reminder: The advice in this book is only for you if you are otherwise fully functioning apart from drinking more than you want. This is often referred to as being a grey area drinker (see Jolene Park's contribution on page 26), and you have probably had periods of being alcohol-free in the past. If you are alcohol dependent – if you need alcohol to get the day going or are on medication or under supervision from Alcohol Services or the equivalent – then please *do not* stop suddenly. This can be extremely dangerous; you must see your doctor.

This book is for you if you want some clarity around why it's a good idea to give up, and you want to live your absolute best life. It's also for you if you want to accelerate your healing and wellbeing after drinking. Most of us are aware that, after years of caning it, our bodies and emotions take time to recalibrate, everything gets shaken up! We will address some of the components that will help to get you in balance and feeling better more quickly. Even if you have been sober for a good while, some of the tips and ideas will benefit you, and open you up to new possibilities.

If you have already stopped drinking, are there other addictions you'd like to crack? The good news is you can use many of the same principles.

Five reasons to do an alcohol-free challenge…and rock it sober.

1. Your body and mind will thank you greatly for a period of detox – 7, 30, 60, 90 days without poison? Yes, please!

2. You will get to experience life in all its technicolour glory. Yes, it does mean you can't 'numb out', but you also get to live life to the full. Hey, you could even regularly enjoy two 6 o'clocks in 1 day!

3. You will save money! Get an app that counts your days and the amount you're saving. Top Tip: be honest about the amount you usually spend on booze and put it into a nice glass jar or vase, or pay it into a separate account, then watch it mount up!

4. You will find yourself with extra time on your hands. You know, all those hours you wasted thinking about drinking – planning it, drinking it, feeling wasted, being hungover. You can use those hours to find a new hobby, connect with your real friends, learn a new skill.

5. You will, in due course, experience some of the many benefits of sobriety: clearer skin, better sex, reduced anxiety, more clarity, deeper connections, regulated weight, better sleep (not for the first few weeks, though!), better finances, having more energy, feeling calmer, feeling braver, and feeling happier (alcohol steals your joy).

Still need persuading that life is better without the booze? Of course, being free from any addiction is a great idea, but I remember back quite clearly to when I knew deep down that I had to stop, but not one bit of me wanted to. I knew instinctively that my life would be better physically and emotionally but I was also terrified I wouldn't succeed. I thought I'd lose all my friends and definitely with them would disappear my mojo and my sparkle.

In fact, as you have heard me say so many times if you listen to the podcast Alcohol Free Life or watched my TEDx talk, Sobriety Rocks – Who Knew! Now I almost don't recognise that person who despite being a relatively smart human being couldn't crack the alcohol habit. I knew about holistic living and ditching the toxins in everything from food to skincare, but wine o'clock had a hold over me and I thought I was the only one! I want you to know that you are not alone, there are so many grey area drinkers – not at rock bottom but definitely not take it or leave it, happy social drinkers. This is amazingly good news! You are not alone in this, and you absolutely can crack it, and you will find as I did what author Catherine Gray calls 'the unexpected joy of being sober'.

So, what is a grey area drinker?

Jolene Park, functional nutritionist, health coach and the founder of Healthy Discoveries, gave a TEDx talk Gray Area Drinking. Here's how she described it:

> Gray area drinking is the space between rock bottom drinking and every now and again drinking. Gray area drinkers have the capacity and ability to stop drinking and they do stop drinking – often many times before they ultimately quit drinking for good. Gray area drinkers will choose to stop drinking for a period of time and then they say to themselves 'I'm not that bad, I can be a social drinker, I don't need to be so restrictive.' However, when they return to drinking, they quickly regret their drinking all over again. This back and forth cycle of stopping and restarting drinking, plus the inner struggle around drinking, is very characteristic of gray area drinkers.

This is the kind of drinking where there's no rock bottom, but you drink as a way to manage anxiety and then regret how much and how often you drink. Regardless of the cause of anxiety or discomfort in your life, and regardless of whether you're using alcohol or another substance or behaviour as an attempt to manage stress, grey area drinking is 'the space between the extremes of rock-bottom drinking and every now and again drinking.'

It's up to you how you use this book to help you. Some people work through the sections across 7 days or 30 days, others take 90 days. Make sure you mark down important milestones – once you have reached 7 days, 30 days, reward yourself with a treat that isn't food or drink!

There are some questions to work through, and I highly recommend that you invest in a lovely new notebook, and a pen you actually enjoy writing with. Of course you can use a laptop, phone, etc too, but you may find you do want to take up the tips around journaling and writing gratitude lists – and writing by hand is good for the cognitive brain. I'd love to hear how you are getting on. As you will see, it's important to tell someone what you are doing, even if it's only me! You can find my contact details at the back of the book, or join The Sober Club, our online membership portal which has a private online community alongside; see www. happyhealthysober.com.

When I finally white-knuckled it through that Dry January, I was blessed to have discovered a whole community who seemed to be saying: Stick with this, life is *better*. I could barely believe it at the time, I thought my life would be over, I believed that it would make me boring. *Sober* is an anagram of *bores*.

Turns out, that couldn't be further from the truth!

Chapter 5
PREPARING TO DITCH THE DRINK

Step 1. The big why

Be honest: why did you invest in this book? Have you found yourself Googling 'Am I drinking too much?' I'm guessing you are not entirely happy with your drinking and you have a suspicion that you would feel better if it stopped.

There's no doubt that addictive substances can have a hold on us. It was a shock to me when I first realised that I – a fairly determined, otherwise relatively bright, successful professional couldn't win over the wine witch and the desire to drink. It came as a shock to me that alcohol is seriously addictive and plays tricks with your mind over time.

It doesn't actually matter how much you are drinking – if it's an issue for you, it's an issue. I'm guessing you saw a glimmer of hope that you too might find the buzz without the booze, that you might be able to lose weight, sleep better, stop waking up not being able to remember what you did or said the night before. You probably want to give up, to experience a life without being addicted to what's in a glass.

But I'm guessing there is also a part of you that probably just wants to be a normal drinker. I'd be rich if I had a pound for every time I said, 'Why can't I just have one, like normal people?' The answer was because I had a voice in my head, an addictive voice compelling me to drink, and after one drink, I didn't have an off switch. Some people can manage to be fully in control of alcohol

– though I will argue, Why do you want to be?. We will talk more about mindful drinking later (see page 103) but for now ...

... go ahead and determine your big **Why.**

In your notebook, ask yourself: ***Why** do I want to be free from booze?*
If you can bear it, recall one experience from your drinking career which you'd rather forget. Perhaps you drank too much and felt terrible the next day, perhaps it got messy with a friend or loved one, maybe you spent more money than you should have. Make it as descriptive as possible, no one else needs to read it, but do write it all down, warts and all. It's the only negative thing I'm going to ask you to do, but please do it. Call it an 'F– off, alcohol' letter if you want.

***Why** do I want to be sober?*

What do you hope ditching the booze will offer you? If you have heard people talk about benefits that you'd like for yourself, write those down. Think of as many reasons as possible for why you'd like to be sober.
Write down all of these thoughts, preferably by hand (it's good for the cognitive brain). Then put it in a sealed envelope addressed to yourself and put it in a safe place.

Now answer the question: ***Why** don't I want to give up?*

You may think this is a trick question, or that I'm being face-tious, but whenever we have an issue in our lives, it's recognized that there is usually some reverse psychology going on, some strong and deep-rooted beliefs which hold us back from achieving what we claim to want.

So grab another piece of paper and write down: ***Why** do I want to carry on the way I am?*

What's stopping me from giving up? Is it the right time? Let's face it, if we keep making excuses there will never feel like a right time. If we wait till the weekend, or after a party, or when we're back from holiday, there will always be more occasions, more reasons. The best time is right now!

Could it be FOMO (fear of missing out) or fear of missing alcohol that's holding your back? That's a common one. Many of us really do believe deep down that all our best times are when alcohol has been present. And if we have been drinking since we were in our teens or early twenties, that may be a long time! Alcohol has literally been our longest meaningful relationship! Of course we are going to be a bit fearful of the first party without it, the first time we have sober sex, the first networking meetings, the first holidays without alcohol – how will we cope? It's natural to feel the fear at the beginning. Accept that feeling.

Answer the question: ***Why*** *are you stopping yourself from giving up?*

Just write with a stream of consciousness, don't edit yourself. You may find you write something like 'I believe that drinking makes me more confident, eases my social anxiety / I won't be able to be creative without drinking [lots of creatives fear that] / I won't get to feel grown-up after a day with the kids.' It might be that you are fearful of upsetting your partner; if they see you as their drinking buddy, could that be an issue?

Whatever it is, be honest and get it all out there.

Next question: *How much am I drinking?* Or: *How much was I drinking before I stopped recently?*

If you are like me, you will be kidding yourself that you drink less than you do. We all know that keeping a food diary when we are trying to diet is agonising, especially having to see in black and white every biscuit, snack and naughty treat – but it does make a difference. Be realistic and write down how much you are drinking – or were drinking if you have recently stopped. No one else needs to know. And remember, whether it's an amount that means you have serious health dangers or not, if it's an issue for you, if it means you are having anything other than your *best* life, then it needs addressing. I sometimes refer to the booze elevator – don't wait till you're at rock bottom before you hop off.

Once you've written down this stuff, take a deep breath! Don't worry about studying what you've written too much. Just be sober curious and file it away in a safe place.

Decide to ditch the booze while you work through this section.

You may have ditched the booze for a while before, but this time it's different. You've decided to commit to this and you are going to write at least 10 lines, about your **Big Why**.

Triggers

To get a true sense of where you are at, think about the triggers that usually cause you to drink.

See if you can recall when you last decided to drink. Of course there may be some obvious ones – you were at a restaurant, at a party – but what about when you drank at home, or if you drank alone, what was it that made you decide to do that? You can use the classic interview questions that we learn when training as an interviewer:

Who? What? When? Where? Why? How?

Who do I usually drink with? Friends, colleagues, family?

What is my choice of drink, and why do I like it?

When do I drink? Evenings, weekends, at gatherings, with meals?

Where do I drink? At home, in pubs, clubs?

Why do I continue to drink, even though I have identified I'd like to slow down or stop?

How much do I really drink? Be honest!

These questions can help you to evaluate how you view alcohol. Do you see it as a reward? A treat? Do you use it to numb your feelings – if so, what feelings in particular? Do you drink because you feel it allows you to relax, to appear more confident? Be your own psychiatrist and ask yourself some hard questions, then write down the honest answers.

How do you usually feel after the first drink? How do you feel after the third or fourth drink?

How does drinking change who you are? Does it make you feel more confident, more outgoing, more able to face the day? Have others ever told you that you seem like a different person when you drink?

What is your social persona? Are you the life and soul of the party, the person who likes a drink?

What about when you are alone with your thoughts? What kind of person are you before you reach for that first glass?

Ask yourself a few general health and wellbeing questions too:

Are you at your ideal weight right now?

Are you generally healthy? If not, what are my main ailments?

Do you sleep well?

Are you anxious?

Where are you on the booze spectrum?

I know you aren't at rock bottom, but you aren't at the top of the booze elevator either, or you wouldn't be reading this! So how far down are you, and how easy is it for you to step off? This is important because it's an elevator that, left to its own mechanics, only goes down. You may feel confident that you would never slip further down into dependent levels of drinking, but who knows what life may throw at you? There have been many people who have found themselves in a situation where they can only reach for the bottle and slide further down.

Get clarity on where you are at now and be committed to your decision as to where you want to be.

33

The real question isn't: *Should I drink a bit less?* or *Should I give up for a while every few months?* or *Should I drink something different with less ABV [alcohol by volume]?*

The **real** question is: *Would my life be better physically and emotionally without alcohol?*

That's a big one, and the answer is often a big fat YES, but it can feel too scary to do anything about it.

Reward time

Once you have written down your thoughts and answered the questions, I want you to give yourself a reward. Don't worry, they don't have to cost a lot (if anything). Your reward is to choose one self-care treat from the list below – and enjoy it!

- Reward yourself with a lovely warm bath with essential oils, or burn oils in a diffuser
- Walk in nature, sit with your back against a tree
- Buy yourself a nice new notebook or journal and pen
- Treat yourself to a bunch of seasonal flowers or a plant
- Make your favourite meal, light a candle and play your favourite music.

Step 2. Make your commitment

You've committed, I hope, to ditch the booze for at least 7 days – or 30 days for real impact. It's a big thing and it might get tough, but you can do it and it's *so* worth it.

Let me be realistic, though. The benefits won't all come at once or straight away. A few people will find themselves more happy, full of energy, sleeping well and at their ideal weight within a week of giving up. Some of these benefits come later to the rest of us, but believe me, they are well worth waiting for.

In case you're still floundering as to whether you are doing the right thing, I'd love to encourage you to discover for yourself a few home truths about alcohol. Have a look at the statistics on alcohol-related problems and illnesses on the Alcohol Change UK websitewww.alcoholchange.org.uk. Another useful source of information is the NHS website: www.nhs.uk/conditions/alcohol-misuse/

It's not stated that alcohol causes mental illness, stress and anxiety, but it most certainly exacerbates these problems. A Lifesearch survey found that 24 million people in the UK admitted to self-medicating with alcohol to ease their anxiety and stress (ironic, as alcohol is a depressant).

Alcohol is not thought of as a Class A drug, yet when other factors are brought into the equation – in other words, not just the harm to the individual but also the harm to others, the economy, the cost to the health service – alcohol comes out top.

Yep, booze is the Number 1 most harmful drug!

Does this help you to be more clear that this decision is going to be for the best for you? It will probably be the single best decision you ever make in your life. Exciting, isn't it!

Remind yourself of the benefits that will come your way. Keep a list – and take it from me, though you may not believe me now, you will come through this. You will feel like a completely different person when you are no longer under the control of your alcohol cravings and addictive thoughts.

Take note of the fabulous phrase and the title of a book by Laura McKowen: *We are the luckiest.*

Time is being called on alcohol in the UK as well as around the world, and it's a trend that's growing rapidly. This is borne out by the massive rise in popularity and demand in alcohol-free and low alcohol drinks. The demand has been met by the big players and producers alongside the artisan breweries and little brands who are making a big difference. There's more later on the great new trends in alcohol-free drinks (see page 105) and do check the Resources section too (page 207).

The media are starting to notice this shift too. It's regularly reported that many more of us are choosing not to drink, or to drink less, and trying one of the sober months such as Dry January or Sober October and not looking back. Of course, if you are ditching the booze, you are in very good company. There are lots of sober celebrities including Zoe Ball, Davina McCall, Bradley Cooper and many more – no doubt that's why they look so good!

It is super important for you to get support on this journey. No one can do it alone. At least, it's much easier with someone to cheer you on and give you some accountability. Get your inspiration any which way too. Read quit lit books and memoirs and find other sober heroes to encourage you on social media.

Check out the reading list (page 201). It's a big help to find someone whose story resonates with yours. For me, in the first few weeks when the chips were down and I felt like reaching for a glass of wine, and struggled to imagine that I'd ever feel differently, it was reading and rereading certain books that really helped me pull through.

Get connected

You may want to attend a group meeting; it can be super powerful to be accountable to a group. Everyone is aware of AA, but there is also SMART Recovery and several other groups. If the idea of joining a group resonates with you, find one near you. If not, don't worry because there are many other ways of meeting others; a social group may work well for you or an online community support may be just the thing. You are very welcome to join me at The Sober Club!

You really don't have to go it alone and that's great news. There's more on getting social later in the book (see Chapter 10), but for now I just want you to know that it's a great idea to step into this, and go for it, to find your people and get connected.

However you are feeling now, the next action step is important.

Tell someone. Make it real

This is a big one. We all need someone rooting for us. You may well not be ready to tell the world, your partner, your family or friends, but tell one person your intentions. Ideally someone who knows you, who you know will be supportive. You can also email me. If you are part of The Sober Club, tell the Facebook group, or tell another group you are part of – but tell someone, to make it real. You may benefit from attending meetings or from connecting with a sober coach to help guide you through. Do what feels right for you, but don't keep it completely to yourself.

Step 3. Get your sober tools ready

Now you've made your commitment and have a clear idea of your why – hopefully, super clear – but you are also aware that it will be at least a bit hard. Anything worth doing is hard, right? But it's not impossible and it's surely made easier when you have laid the foundations and have your sober tools in place.

What are your sober tools? The resources, the tips, the tricks, the snacks, the phrases, the apps, the support you need to ensure that you stay on track.

Remember, this is non-negotiable! You have made a decision and you are going to stick with it. Here is a technique that will help you stay on track of your progress and motivated:

The WOOP technique

This approach is known as Mental Contrasting, and was developed by Dr Gabriele Oettingen. It has been used effectively in many areas of life and is a great planning tool for changing behaviour. It's great to use it regularly to keep yourself accountable. WOOP stands for: Wish; Outcome; Obstacle; Plan.

Wish   a feasible goal, a meaningful challenge.
           Set your wish, and make it a memorable phrase.
Outcome   what is the outcome you want? What is the best result
           or feeling from accomplishing that wish?
           Ask yourself how you will feel when you succeed.
           Remind yourself of some of the rewards you are looking
           forward to.
Obstacle   what is within you that might prevent you from accom-
           plishing your wish?
           Be honest about what might crop up to make you feel
           wobbly.

37

Plan   what will be your plan of action if the obstacle presents itself?

What action will be effective?

Hopefully you have already identified what you want (to ditch the booze) and the outcome you want (perhaps to sleep better, to have more energy, to be free from addiction). You have probably identified the reasons you may not want to give up – i.e. maybe you are afraid that you will feel ridiculous telling others you don't drink. So what's the plan? How will you prepare for when/if that happens? You might decide on a good response, and get a couple of supportive people on your side.

Let's suppose your *Wish* is to ditch the booze for 7 days or 30 days. Your *Outcome* may be that you know you will feel lighter, happier and proud of yourself, and that you will be looking forward to saving enough money for a day trip to the seaside. Your *Obstacle* might be that you always have friends over for drinks at the end of the month – and that's got you worried. *Plan* to create an innovative mocktail evening, get some great recipes and be inspired by some great new drinks that everyone will love.

Write down your WOOP on a piece of paper and keep it where you can see it. Make a note of it on your phone and use the technique every time you have a new situation coming up.

Make your commitment now!

Tracking your progress

If you haven't yet get yourself an app that counts your sober dates, enter into it the date you stopped. Then make a note of what you used to spend daily on alcohol, and watch this rack up. Choose an app such as I Am Sober which shows days, time and money saved.

Buy or find a nice glass jar and put that money into it. If you usually use a credit card to pay for booze (seems less that way!), make sure you actually draw the cash out of the bank and stash it in the jar, at least for a few weeks; you will be amazed how it racks up. Either way, watch that app as it climbs up and be proud of yourself.

'I am 748 days in, saved £7,480, learned lots along the way and will never go back!!'

Alison

It's amazing how much Alison has saved by counting the days and the amount she would have spent if she was still drinking over this period of time.

Counting the days is a big one. Celebrate when you hit 7 days, 30 days and each milestone. And of course I mean treat yourself with something that's actually a treat. (For inspiration, look at the self-care list, page 34). Isn't it bizarre how we are all so conditioned that it's hard to say the word *celebrate* without thinking of a glass of bubbly?

Chapter 6
BREAKING THE HABIT.
THE FIRST 7 DAYS

To begin with, there can be quite a lot to navigate.

Maybe stopping drinking is simple for you. You may suffer with a headache for a few days, then feel OK. Or you may find this much more difficult to do. If you've been off the booze for a few days, you might feel like you are on an emotional roller coaster.

However, you feel, understand that this is perfectly normal! I felt really quite raw for the first few weeks, and over time had to get used to a whole new way of being.

Here are some tips for your first 7 days:

- Find something to keep you busy, fill your time, change the routine of your day or evening – especially the times when you will crave that drink!
- Eat well and ensure you have the right nutrition.
- Make sure you have a healthy alternative to drinking when the craving hits. Chocolate is the obvious one. If you have a sweet tooth, it is likely you will crave sweet foods. Buy yourself the best raw, organic, high percentage cacao chocolate. Organic dates are good too for when you get the sweet munchies. Or, if you can resist the sweet stuff, keep healthy snacks to hand.

- Drink plenty of water. A lovely water bottle, or a reusable bottle, is good to have with you to take your favourite drinks in when you are out and about.
- A notebook can be an amazing sober tool. Have a go at journaling. Literally write your thoughts down, don't edit or judge. It's a stream of consciousness and you may be surprised what you write down. Each evening, write down a list of things you are grateful for. This is so simple but can be so profound; you may have had a tricky day, but you can always find things to be grateful for. Start with at least three things each day.
- Try something digital. An app to count your progress or keep you connected to your online groups and friends.
- Find inspiration – podcasts on sobriety, hypnosis audios and meditations, quit lit books.
- Try something academic – read books or research papers, listen to talks on the psychology of addiction, discover what alcohol really is.
- Do something social – physical meet-ups, sober social events, online communities.
- Here are the changes Vicky put in place to make it easier.

My one tip that worked for me was: distraction. For the first few months, I had to do a U-turn on my evening routine which had previously consisted of going to the pub with mates and picking up wine on the way home. My wine witch usually started badgering me as I was finishing work. To combat her, I started running during the evenings and swerving visits to the pub. I created barriers at home to stop me from nipping out to the off-licence, such as washing my hair when I got back from work and changing straight into pyjamas. I think, for those who were drinking as heavily as I was, you have to really throw yourself into the world of not drinking.

The public perception of quit lit has shifted and I think it's more socially acceptable to be reading books about self-improvement.

Vicky

When you've made it to day 7, your first week of sobriety, make sure you give yourself a reward. You could download a film or have a candle-lit bubble bath. Treat yourself to something that makes you feel good.

Let's also have a quick recap!

What has been the hardest part of this week for you? What were the trigger points that made you nearly give in? How did you deal with them?

Were you able to focus on something to do that did not involve you drinking? Did you go for a walk or coffee with a friend? Did you do something for yourself that you haven't done in ages?

Did you implement the WOOP technique?
Have you identified your Wish, the Outcome you want? What the Obstacle might be? Did you make your Plan?

Perhaps you tripped up and drank against your own better judgement. I'm purposely not calling that a 'relapse' because I don't think it's helpful. If you had a setback, see it just as that – a setback, a trip-up – and you can start all over again. Most of us are way too hard on ourselves. When we are dieting, we don't usually give up completely if we stray from our plan, but when we come to quitting alcohol we want perfection. Having said that, I'm not giving you carte blanche to keep drinking whenever the thoughts come in!

The important question to ask is: Why did you trip up? We do know that no one falls over a drink and consumes it. So when you look back, dig deep into what happened. Did you choose to have that drink because something else was really going on? Were you upset about something, scared, or were you actually hungry?

For every day you didn't drink, did you congratulate yourself? Are you using your sober app and counting days?

Have you listened to any podcast episodes? Have you read any inspirational quit lit?

Did you tell someone what you are doing?

I hope you managed to tell someone, even if it was only me! I'm going to keep rubbing it in: as Johann Hari says, the opposite of addiction is connection. You may not feel like being ultra-social yet, but let someone know. You need support and if you know you have told at least one person, your subconscious mind will remind you if you feel triggered to drink, that you'll have to tell them.

Did you experience cravings and triggers?

We will explain cravings next, but triggers come in different forms and are different for different people. Cravings are just thoughts, and we can learn to tame them, but usually a trigger comes before that craving, or thought. A sunny day, for example, can trigger the thought of sitting outside in a pub garden drinking a cool drink. Of course, your rational brain knows that the drink could be anything – a sparkling water, an alcohol-free beer, a mocktail – but the thoughts can quickly turn into feelings which you associate with drinking, and you might feel strongly that you want to experience the 'numbing out' which alcohol can provide. The trick is to challenge the trigger and look at what the feelings around it are.

It's quite a thing retraining your brain, and forming new habits, but we now know it can be done. We can form new neural pathways in the brain and literally start over till the new ways become automatic. When you get into a new car, or someone else's car and the indicator is on the other side of the steering wheel, you may find yourself reaching for the indicator lever and hitting the wipers instead, or vice versa. You may even berate yourself for not getting it yet, but over time and with repeated correction of the behaviour you learn the new way, and that soon becomes the default setting.

Chapter 7
THE NEXT 30 DAYS!

I want you to focus on all the positive benefits of continuing to not drink.

Once you'd stopped drinking, the physical cravings will almost certainly have abated within the first few days. The alcohol is gone, so after the first a few days any irritation and discomfort you are feeling is in your head. That doesn't mean it's insignificant – cravings are the worst – but when you realise that it's just your mind up to tricks, you'll be better equipped to deal with it.

Understanding cravings

Let's talk more about cravings and look at what they really are.

William Porter, author of *Alcohol Explained*, describes this well. He says that cravings are just thoughts. Pretty powerful ones, but just thoughts.

Many of us are aware of the addictive voice in our head. We sometimes call it the wine witch, she often flies in at around wine o'clock and says: 'Go on, you deserve a treat, you can just have one.' It's the addictive voice in our head that tells us to finish the bottle, to plan to be at the cinema or wherever we are going early to have time to get a drink; it's this voice that tells us we *need* the alcohol. That nudges us toward reading the copious amounts of media coverage driven by the alcohol industry which tell us that alcohol is good for us. We love it when we hear stories of people who drink way more than we do who lived into their nineties.

Jack Trimpey, a former social worker in the United States, is the author of the brilliant book *Rational Recovery: The New Cure for Substance Addiction*. Jack developed a whole programme, AVRT (Additive Voice Recognition Technique) and it was a major breakthrough in recovering from substance addiction. He believes that if you can acknowledge and tame the addictive voice, you can take responsibility for your own path and make a full recovery. I definitely had that addictive voice, it compelled me to drink yet another glass of wine. It's good to know it's been written about, it's a 'thing'!

Of course, this all tracks back to the power of the mind. Our subconscious mind is very clever at protecting us, it likes us to do what we have always done. It's not possible to be addicted to anything unless we experience some kind of pleasure or reward from it. When alcohol seemed to be the missing piece – when we found that suddenly as a shy teenager we could feel confident after a drink, or when we found that networking meetings seemed so much more glamorous with a drink in the hand – we made those associations in the brain. Don't forget our subconscious mind doesn't make value judgements, it recognises the facts: drink taken = feeling relaxed, chilled, happy.

Therefore, it will constantly seek out more of those feelings and if they have always been associated with alcohol, the 'addictive voice' within will continue to demand that we drink.

Of course, this is all just a big old fight going on inside our head, but it's important to remember that our thoughts create our feelings, and that it's our feelings, our emotions that lead to the actions we take.

When you crave alcohol, be conscious of the thoughts and ask yourself what's really going on. Check in with the acronym **HALT – Hungry, Angry, Lonely, Tired.**

When you feel you really want to reach for a drink, are you in fact:

Hungry? Sometimes you just need to eat, it's a blood sugar problem. Think carefully about having good snacks to hand.

Angry? Are you actually feeling fed up about anything? When you are feeling angry, emotions spiral and the misconception is that alcohol will help. Instead ask yourself what's making you angry. Sometimes it's therapeutic to take yourself off somewhere private and scream and shout for a while, or punch a cushion!

Lonely? Loneliness is not fun. As humans we want to feel connected. If you are feeling lonely, you won't find friendship in a bottle. Loneliness can be a big one when you first change your relationship with alcohol, because we link alcohol to being social, and not drinking when with friends makes it's easy to feel a bit isolated.

Try to make contact with someone who is going through the same emotions. The Sober Club and other online groups have become so important in helping people with similar issues connect with each other. Make plans to attend some meetings or at least join some sober communities. Find your tribe!

Tired? Somehow, we have managed to convince ourselves that if we are exhausted a drink will help. It definitely won't. If you have been overdoing it, or if you feel tired, give your body what it needs: sleep. Who cares if it's only 7 p.m.? If it's possible, get into your PJs, take a herbal tea and sleep. If it's not possible, then find a way of relaxing; listen to a meditation tape or relax in a warm bath.

How the craving brain works

Have you come across the fantastic analogy of the elephant, the rider and the path? It can be really helpful for understanding why otherwise bright people have such a struggle changing their habits. It's courtesy of Professor Jonathan Haidt.

Imagine a big elephant with someone sitting on his back. The elephant represents your emotional brain; at its front is the amygdala, which is the part that responds to stress and fear. The rider sitting on top of the elephant represents you – holding the reins and driving your emotional brain. It seems at first glance that control lies with you, the rider because you can lead the elephant where you want it to go. In fact, the elephant is huge and unwieldy, so if something sets off a stress response or a strong emotion in the elephant, it will take off in a different direction – and however much you the rider want to try and head down a new path, that isn't going to happen if the elephant doesn't feel safe or comfortable!

When I am teaching people to be great public speakers or give presentations, I try to drive this home:

Emotions, not logic, inspire action

What I mean by that is we can all be given reams and reams of logical information. We can learn facts and statements and accept and believe on a rational level that we should operate a certain way. Over the years I'm sure we have all read and digested thoroughly the statistics around alcohol and the harms it brings. But however powerful those awful truths are, they haven't resulted in many of us ditching the booze. Why? Because our subconscious mind, our elephant, associates drinking with doing what we have always done, with feeling rewarded, relaxed, chilled, with being social and sociable. Intrinsically our inner elephant definitely doesn't want to branch out down a new unknown path that feels very scary and definitely worse.

> *I hate having feelings. Why does sobriety have to come with feelings? One minute I feel excited, the next I feel terrified. One minute I feel free and the next I feel doomed.*
>
> Augusten Burroughs

The path represents where we are headed and our environment. Typically, the elephant and our subconscious mind want to go where we always go, down the path of least resistance. We don't want a struggle between the rider and the elephant, it never turns out well!

So what's the answer here? Well, if emotions and not logic inspire the action, we need to seek out the positive emotions. When we can see the light at the end of the tunnel and it seems bright and wonderful, that will evoke a happy feeling which means our subconscious mind will be happy to give it a try.

If we have recognised that drinking mocktails, for example, will mean we will be feeling happy and bright and ready to head off out early the next morning, that's a good feeling and both elephant and rider are happy to go to the bar and opt for a virgin mojito. But there are still some potential obstacles to overcome. If we have planned to go out with colleagues who will challenge our decision not to drink, and we haven't thought through how we will answer them when they give us a hard time, that will create conflict – and it could be that the elephant caves in under the duress and leads us back on the wrong path.

At this point, it's not about facts or reason, it's about emotions. So we need to remember our Big Why and then be ready to break it down into specifics. It's not enough to say: 'I'm not drinking ever again.' Goodness knows we've all said that a million times when hungover. We need to have really made our decision on an emotional level and really embody and imagine the outcome.

Some people need to think right back to how they were as children before they 'needed' alcohol to have fun. If you stop drinking and feel any kind of benefit, write that down and fully embrace it. The more positive emotional references you can build up, the greater your capacity to guide your elephant in the best direction and motivate it. When it comes to the environment, it may not all be within your control, but you can plan ahead. We will deal later with how to handle friends in social situations (see Chapter 10), but at the very least plan where you are going, with whom and how you will handle the tricky questions.

Having success over cravings and changing habits is about introducing a series of new habits. Focus on the successful, positive ones.

When it comes to the path, this really relates to cravings. The environment you are in, will affect the thoughts you have, and this in turn will affect your feelings – and as we know, emotions inspire action.

So when cravings strike, and they will – of course they will – try and calmly remember: *It's just a thought.* Granted, it will feel very persuasive: *I need a drink, I* deserve *a drink.* Rather than do what you have always done, pause and ask yourself:

What is it that I really want/need right now?

A craving can be like an annoying 'itch' that needs to be scratched, but perhaps it can be relieved a different way

Ask yourself: Is it true that I 'need' alcohol?

Of course not!

Is it really a treat?

No, definitely not.

A walk in nature, a lovely soak in a bath with essential oils, a warming drink of chocolate, that's a treat – but not a glass of fermented liquid. So get into the habit of challenging your own thoughts, and if the cravings are strong, pay it forward. Imagine how you will feel tomorrow morning if you cave in now and finish the bottle of wine. Chances are you will remember that you will feel hungover, and miserable that you let yourself down.

You absolutely can work with the elephant. Decide together to choose the best path because you are having happy positive thoughts.

Often, when we are trying to change habits, we are focusing on what we *can't* have. This obviously upsets our elephant and makes us feel hard done by, and deprived. It's far better, with your determined Big Why in mind, to think about what you can have. Of course you can have alcohol, but you are choosing not to.

> ... I could if I wanted, have a glass of wine, but I haven't had one because I really haven't wanted one! Wow! The stroppy toddler or teenager in me just didn't want to be told I couldn't! And I'm loving it. Seven months have gone by so quickly and I'm so much clearer in my head. The fog has lifted. I left the shore, paddled backwards a few times and I'm determined and happy to go forward and reach the other side.
>
> Karen S

So what can you have that makes you feel good? Herbal tea, an alcohol-free drink, kombucha, hot chocolate? The list is endless. Or it may be that you don't need to consume anything at all. Instead, scratch the itch – by going for a walk, dancing, doing some exercise, reading a book.

Reward yourself with at least one fun thing.

Taming the sugar monster

We will talk later in this book about good nutrition and the important foods for you to focus on (see Chapter 14), but first I want to address the issue that affects so many people, the fact that when you quit the booze it's common to crave – or think you crave – sugar. People say that once they stop drinking, the ice cream and chocolate is literally calling them. It's normal but can be very annoying, especially if you're hoping to get healthier and lose weight. It's very common to transfer an alcohol addiction to a sugar addiction. Of course, since childhood most of us have been taught to believe that sugar is a treat. We have a lot emotionally invested in sugar, so when we first give up alcohol, which for many of us was our treat, we often think we should reward ourselves with copious amounts of chocolate and sweets.

We're often told that alcohol is full of sugar. Because some grapes are not so ripe, some wines have sugar added during fermentation too. For this reason, some people suggest drinking spirits which don't contain sugar, but remember that a mixer such as tonic water will contain sugar.

The bottom line is that most of us have had biochemical stuff going on for a long time. What I mean is that many people who find themselves over-drinking or addicted to cigarettes or drugs have got biochemical deficiencies. Neurotransmitters are the feel-good brain chemicals, and many of us are out of balance. Sometimes the reason we have been reaching for yet another drink is because we are feeling out of whack, anxious or stressed. We reach for a drink, which at least initially gives us that boost of serotonin or GABA, helping our mood. But sadly, it's temporary and while we might feel that initial buzz and improved mood and a sense of *ah ... now*

I can relax, that's quickly followed by restless sleep and all kinds of other alcohol-induced issues.

So it stands to reason that if you are someone who is deficient in some of these neurotransmitters and it feels normal to reach for substances to help, then it's likely that if you've decided you won't reach for alcohol, the next in line will be sugar.

Just like alcohol, sugar can temporarily raise these chemicals in the body. We all know the expression 'sugar rush', and sugar along with caffeine can also raise those serotonin levels, albeit temporarily.

You may also have issues with blood sugar levels, and this is one area where you can try and take back some control.

Keep the ritual, change the ingredients

There are, of course, some more healthy ways of getting your sugar fix. For starters, mix up your styles of sugar: try having a spoonful of honey, a drizzle of maple syrup, pop an organic medjool date in the freezer – yum, it tastes a bit like a rich chocolate, really hits the spot. Grapes in the freezer are great too. Teach yourself to make some simple healthy sweet treats. Get some fruit, then whizz it in a blender and freeze it. Or blend frozen berries, add a few chopped nuts and chia seeds and, voilà, a fabulous sweet frozen yoghurt dessert.

If you love chocolate, you're definitely quids in; proper chocolate is actually good for you. Of course, high percentage cacao isn't sweet at all and needs something added, but experiment with making raw chocolate desserts.

Just one word of warning, though. Don't be tempted in your quest to avoid sugar to opt for artificial sweeteners: these synthetic chemicals are literally the last thing you need when you are already potentially deficient in mood-boosting brain chemicals; they have been defined as neurotoxins and banned in some countries. Never opt for a diet drink. If sugar is bad, artificial sweeteners are worse.

A teaspoon of apple cider vinegar may help with the cravings. And to ensure that you are getting some great nutrients, a handful of pumpkin seeds might do the trick: add a few to porridge oats with some cinnamon for a healthy sugar craving buster!

Putting in the good nutrition

You know how most of us fib if we're asked how much we drink by our GP? Well, most of us fib about what we eat too. We would hate to be asked to keep a food diary and have to write down absolutely everything we eat. If asked about our diet, we often say 'Oh, I eat fairly healthily, lots of salads and fruit, brown rice etc', but the reality is lots of us find that days go by and we have really not had our quota of fresh fruit and veg,

The optimum amount is meant to be 5 portions of fruit and veg per day, but I'd argue that we need closer to 10. Health and nutrition is covered in more detail in Part 2. A reminder of the basics of good nutrition is never more important for you than when you are changing your habits around alcohol.

When I quit drinking, I forgot to drink enough water! Tip: fill up a large bottle and drink from it throughout the day. Or just drink lots of tea! Builders, herbal or infusions will do. Organic and caffeine free is best, though.

Hippocrates said, *'Let food be they medicine, and medicine be they food.'*

So true! If you feed your body the right fuel, you will work your way to optimum health and wellbeing, and that's how you have energy and vitality whatever your age. Often when people are ditching the booze, they are trying to lose weight too. This is definitely not a good time to be trying to diet! Your priority right now is to get the booze out of the house and the food in!

Chapter 8
CHECKING IN

To keep moving forward once you have made the decision to ditch the booze, and to upscale your life to have more optimum health and wellbeing, it's worth getting to the bottom of why you ended up drinking too much in the first place. Focus on the psychological issues.

Ask yourself the important question: What's underneath it all?

There's no doubt that when you finally ditch the booze it helps enormously with anxiety, but that's not to say that all mental health issue are instantly resolved; that would be too simplistic. It's really important to remember that there is probably a reason, albeit a subconscious one, that you started over-drinking. Initially it was probably just the one thing, but somewhere along the line your subconscious mind probably decided that you could benefit from having another and another; there was an itch that the alcohol scratched. You may not be aware of it, or drinking may literally just be a habit, but if you are aware that you were drinking to take a break from some kind of trauma, or because it made your forget something that was hard to deal with, then it's important to realise that those stressors or emotions haven't gone away. Drinking doesn't solve anything, it just gives you temporary relief. We used alcohol for the buzz, it numbs us out for a while, enabling us to step away from our overactive minds and worrying thoughts.

The relief really is temporary, and the result is usually chaos, but for some of us we have been covering up unwanted feelings and emotions for years by anaesthetising ourselves with booze. When the mask comes off, you have to be super grown-up and ask yourself: 'Am I now ready to face this and deal with this another way?'

Identifying the issue is part way to solving it. Be super honest and seek the help you need. You may already feel intuitively that it's right for you to seek therapy, counselling or some kinds of functional medicine treatment.

In one of my podcasts, author Lisa Smith said that it was only once she had sought treatment for her addiction that she got a diagnosis for clinical depression, she had been masking her symptoms for such a long time. Of course, for many people it really is the case that alcohol helped them to feel more confident or able to cope, but do be willing to face the issues head-on. The really great news is that with a few weeks of not drinking under your belt, the bad stuff may not have gone away, but you will definitely be feeling clearer, more resilient and more able to deal with it.

Some people started drinking when they were teenagers. If this is the case for you, it may be that alcohol has been your longest 'meaningful' relationship; it means that all of the big life experiences have been seen through a lens of booze – relationships, sex, fun, holidays, career, *everything*. So it's no wonder that when many of us we take the alcohol away we can be floundering for a while, feeling very ungrounded and out of sorts. All kinds of fluctuating emotions surface in the first weeks and months of sobriety, so don't be at all surprised if this happens for you. I ricocheted from feeling shaky, angry, guilty and a bit depressed to feeling a sense of elation that I'd managed 30 days. Without doubt it was a roller coaster of feelings and emotions

If you know you have lots of underlying issues, I recommend you work with a practitioner. Therapeutic treatments can all help, but it may be that you would benefit from having some sessions with a counsellor or psychotherapist. Don't put this off, seek the help you need. I'm also a big fan of Family Constellations: check out my podcast on this work, sometimes called Homeopathy for the Soul.

Chapter 9
SELF-CARE, SLEEP, RELAXATION, EXERCISE

It's likely that you may experience some issues with your sleep in the first stages of giving up. I hoped that I'd be sleeping like a baby by Day 4. It was not to be. I had pretty disrupted sleep for a good while, but trust me it's worth waiting for. We all know that drinking too much can send us to sleep, but it's not a sleep with much quality; it's usually fitful and we wake during the night or early hours of the morning thirsty and with a racing heartbeat and hating ourselves for doing it all over again. All things being equal, proper restorative sleep will come back to you. Here are a few tips, though, to ensure you help it along.

Firstly, in the early stages, or however long it takes for you, let your bed be your refuge. Treat yourself to whatever you need to feel safe and cosseted in your bed – a new pillow perhaps, some pyjamas, a new dressing gown; it doesn't matter, just make your bed somewhere you want to be. Ideally the room should not be too warm, and here's the big one: ideally no electronic devices. Don't do that thing where you wake yourself with your phone. Ideally, leave it out of the bedroom, but if you have to have it in there, or if you are listening to podcasts – there, broke my own rule, of course I want you to listen to my podcast, or a hypnotherapy tape or similar – then at least turn it to airplane mode when you sleep. If possible, turn off your Wi-Fi too. In the early stages if sleep alludes you, don't lie there stressing about it. Get up for a while and potter about, make a herbal tea and read a book, but don't switch on the news or answer emails – or the whole spiral starts again.

There are some great hypnotherapy audios which can help with sleep, and EFT (emotional freedom techniques, see page 123) can help too.

If you are really struggling to sleep, first try the natural stuff first. Sleep-inducing foods include banana, lettuce, and turkey (it contains tryptophan) and consider herbal remedies, such as drinking chamomile tea, taking valerian root, putting a few drops of lavender oil on your pillow. But if nothing works, seek help.

Resting and relaxation during the day are hugely important too. Many people swear by a good old-fashioned nap in the middle of the day – a power nap as it's been called. I find it impossible, but I do benefit from just lying down for a few minutes. Just allowing your body to rest on the floor, or a mat or even a bed sends a signal to the brain that you are not in panic mode, that it's OK to rest. In the early weeks you may find you feel ridiculously tired. Give in to it, whenever you can.

We spend so much of our lives in a state of urgency. When we are feeling stressed, we're in fight or flight mode, hardwired to get ready to fight or flee from the tiger chasing us ... but actually there are no wild animals, we usually aren't in any immediate danger. Even so, the stress still seems very real. It's really important to find a way to allow our bodies to come out of that urgent state, otherwise we're running on adrenaline, all the time and it's not sustainable.

Sometimes it's enough just to focus on breathing. Of course we do it naturally, but we don't often give it the attention it deserves. Practise a simple breathing technique and it could be transformational: Breathe in through the nose smoothly and effortlessly for a count of 6 seconds, then breathe out through the nose for 6 seconds. You can use simple breathing techniques to calm you down if you're feeling stressed.

Do make sure you work with your body. Some people find that they develop a new habit for exercise but whether you were already moving your body or not, this is the time to ensure that you become aware of the importance of movement. It really is a case of 'use it or lose it', and exercising is one of the quickest cheapest and most natural ways of putting back the feel-good chemicals.

Many people start running – that's not for me, though I never say never – but walking is also great. Basically, the best exercise for you is the one you will do every day. If you're new to exercise, start small. Do a 10-minute walk, then up it to 20 minutes, or move along to some exercise videos. A friend of mine has started lifting weights in her seventies and swears by it! You don't need to join a gym, grab yourself some of those resistance bands and follow some routines on YouTube.

For some people, swimming is amazing. Or put in place some interval training, join a rowing club, go rock climbing. Dancing is amazing; I love Nia dance and also Fitsteps, which is *Strictly* without a partner.

Of course, yoga is brilliant because it's beneficial for mindset too, Pilates can be fantastic for strengthening your core, and ballet is not just for kids; ballet lessons if you can find them near you are fantastic for toning up. If you want to feel like a kid, try rebounding; it's gone out of fashion a bit lately but it's great fun. Just get a mini trampoline, and jump around to your heart's content; it's very safe, as you don't actually put too much pressure on the joints, and you can put on your favourite music.

The bottom line is just move!

Self-care is a big one. If you've listened to any of my podcasts you will know that I bang on about self-care a lot. This is because those of us who spent way too many years drinking way too much alcohol are notoriously bad at proper self-care. We probably used to think we *were* doing OK. If you'd asked me, I would probably have said, 'I'm great at self-care, I give myself a treat of a nice large glass of wine to relax at the end of a busy day. Or I love having a bath with some candles and a nice glass of wine'. All of our perceptions around self-care revolved around the idea of a treat, and that alcohol was it.

Real self-care is asking what you need to nourish yourself physically and emotionally – and it may well not involve consuming anything. Self-care can be as simple as learning to say no if you don't want to go out with friends who are drinking, buying yourself a really nice notebook and writing a gratitude list, it may be having your hair done or booking a spa day, but it may just be as simple as taking a bath, or walking in nature or playing a board game. Pets are brilliant for self-care, so borrow a dog if you don't have one and experience some unconditional love for a while. Get back in touch with what you liked to do as a child. Most of us, caught up in the minutia of adult life, have actually forgotten how to have fun.

Chapter 10
GETTING SOCIAL – HOW TO DEAL WITH RELATIONSHIPS AND THE SOCIAL SCENE

> *Alcohol is the only drug you have to justify not taking.*
>
> Jason Vale

I t is incredibly annoying that the words *social, celebration* and to some extent *fun* have become so intrinsically linked with alcohol. It's actually an illusion; alcohol is just a fermented liquid, not a magic bullet for a great time. But somehow over the years we have all been brainwashed into thinking that it's not possible to be social or to celebrate without a glass of something alcoholic in our hand, and that anyone who isn't imbibing is missing out. This fear of missing out (FOMO) is what stops many people from quitting the booze. We are worried that we won't have fun ever again, we won't be able to laugh, joke, dance and make sparkling conversation without the drink to lubricate everything. In fact, booze really isn't the glue that sticks everything together, and once we can start to see this more clearly we realise that we can have so much more fun and happiness without it! We can eventually reach JOMO (joy of missing out) enjoying what you are doing in each moment without worrying about what everyone else in doing.

At some point when you are feeling a bit more stable, it will feel time to head off out again into the great wide open. Some people rock straight back into the social scene and don't skip a beat; others hole up for a good few weeks while they get their head around their new persona. This is one area where it has to feel right for you. What is important is that you do your preparation. Prepare for your first social outings where alcohol will be present with military precision. It will get easier the more you do it, but at first treat it with respect and remember your Number 1 priority is to protect your sobriety! You've heard the expression 'play the tape forward'; you are definitely not going to feel happy if you allow one weak moment when a mate says: 'Go on, have one' to spoil your however many weeks or months of abstinence.

So do your prep. Firstly, decide if you want to do whatever it is; really think about it. When I look back, I can't believe how much time I wasted hanging around long after the evening had run its natural course, drinking and having – frankly, boring, booze-filled conversations. Once you are sober, you will probably find that you just don't want to stay out as late. Be willing to say no if you don't want to go, it's your prerogative and part of good self-care is setting boundaries. If it's an event or a gathering you do want to go to, or you feel it's not something you can get out of, then plan, plan, plan.

Plan ahead as to what you will drink (more on that later), plan what you will say to friends and others when they ask why you aren't drinking, and plan how you will get home and at what time.

The latter is the easy one. If you drive, there's your get-out clause right there. If you don't want to make a big deal, then your choice not to drink is just that you're driving. But do be careful that you don't just become a free taxi for all your mates; that won't be great self-care! If you are booking yourself a taxi or taking public transport, plan ahead what time that will be and ensure that you don't have to stay longer than you want.

In terms of how you deal with others, that could be the subject for half a book. There are many ways of deflecting comments from others, but again it comes down to planning. If you head off feeling a bit jittery and without having planned, you will probably find yourself stumbling when you are asked about not drinking. Prepare in advance how you want to handle the questions. Some people tell their friends ahead of time, give a heads-up, perhaps by text: 'Hiya, just to let you know I'm off the booze, so more for you!' Or you may want to add: 'I'm not drinking alcohol so would love your support in that decision.'

As yesterday was my Day 100, I decided to 'come out' on Instagram to family and friends. I was so nervous about being so vulnerable, being so honest and 100% me, but guess what??? Comments have been so supportive. Glad I did it and got it over with... I'm hoping it'll open the door for conversations and connection with anyone who's curious about ditching the booze.

T

There will be people who hassle you and ask tricky questions. Often these are the people who probably have their own stuff going on with alcohol, so be strong and unwavering in your decision.

Most friends, if they really are your friends, will support your decision. It is up to you what your chosen response is when they ask. Some people come straight out with 'I feel so much better when I don't drink, it really helps with my anxiety'. Others make a joke: 'I've drunk enough in the last few years, I need to leave some for others.' Some people tell a white lie and say 'I'm on medication' or 'I have an allergy'. Of course, saying you're pregnant works a treat, but can cause all manner of other complications – and clearly won't work for everyone! My point is, decide in advance how you will handle the questions from people who have been socialising with you before when you were drinking.

If it's someone new, they usually won't question it. If I offer someone a drink and they ask for a Coke, it's none of my business. A great response when a work colleague says: 'Would you like a drink?' is to answer in the affirmative, something along the lines of 'Yes, thanks, I'd love a sparkling water'. You don't need to explain, 'Actually I'm not drinking.'

Here's the really good news. In just about every case, this fear that you will be challenged is one that doesn't really occur for many people – at least, not for long. After the initial raised eyebrows or whatever, it's forgotten very quickly. By the time they themselves are onto their second drink, they genuinely couldn't care less what's in your glass.

We will look at some options for said glasses but just a word about relationships outside of the bar. There's nothing like one partner ditching the drink to really shake up a relationship, and how your partner feels about you giving up will probably be a factor in how easy it all is for you. If your partner has been your drinking buddy for ever and a day, this is gonna hit him or her hard. Again, people handle it differently: some focus on themselves and almost hide their sobriety from their partner, others tell their partner just how hard it is for them in the hope that they will be sensitive and offer support. Ultimately this decision is for you: it's your choice, your health and you have to do this for you. It can cause upsets, I won't deny it. I have heard of people who have had to give up on a relationship because this drove them apart. I've also heard many stories of people who quietly got on with their quitting, came out the other side sparkling and stronger and their relationship was all the better for it. The end result will come down to self-care. We lead by our example: I know several sober influencers whose partners decided over time to give up as well, mine included – that was a momentous day when he agreed to purge the house of all the dusty old bottles of booze!

If you are one of the many young people choosing not to drink and on the dating scene, or perhaps it's your second time around, that can be a tough one. The best advice I've heard is from a young woman who said she does give her date a heads-up, letting them know that she is a non-drinker. Most are curious but it doesn't put them off. One guy, she said, did call time on the date – well thank goodness, that saved everyone's time!

Sober sex? That's a big one. Many people may never have had sober sex, ever. Think about that, it's a sobering thought. No wonder many people feel really fearful when there's nothing to ease the awkwardness or increase the confidence. Sometimes it's a case of being patient; if your partner loves you, they will wait while you find yourself again. Literally that's what it feels like, getting sober is coming back to who you really are.

For menopausal women, the whole sex thing can be a big factor in sobriety, at a time when the libido might be dwindling anyway and this creates one hell of a roller coaster of messed-up hormones and brain chemicals. It's really worth seeing a naturopath or nutritional therapist because there could easily be something else going on that's affecting your mood and sexuality aside from just not drinking alcohol.

In terms of getting social, it's not just partners, of course. Your family can cause all kinds of angst. If you come from a family who use alcohol as their social glue, you are going to have to be strong and state your position. If you think your family will make it difficult for you, avoid them for a while. That may sound harsh, but, in my view, you should protect your sobriety at all costs. Make sure you plan ahead and take your own drinks to any occasion. It all comes back to your commitment, so don't let comments or quips from family members or friends rain on your parade.

Getting sober could lead you into a whole new social scene – there's definitely lots available on social media. While it's great to connect with other sober people online, there's no substitute for meeting other people with a shared interest in person. I was hugely nervous when I went along to my first lunch organised by Club Soda. I walked around outside like a kid on her first day at school, but I needn't have worried; everyone was very normal and it was great to discuss shared experiences. It has never been easier to be sober and social. There are meet-ups, lunches, sober raves such as Morning Gloryville, sober bars and even sober karaoke. There are sober dating apps and all kinds of activities for sober millennials and sober singles. There are holidays aimed at people who are sober, and if you are thinking: *Hold on there's nothing in my area*, then start something!

If you can get to London, I regular host events and would love to see you there.

Chapter 11
SOBER DRINKING

What's been great for me is still having lots of treat drinks. I genuinely do deserve something nice to drink at the end of a day, every day, just before I start cooking dinner for the family. So I pour myself a glass of something delicious and visually appealing. I'm actually putting more effort into my drinking and drinking a greater variety than I ever did before. These drinks are my reward for hard work, and they also are the signal to relax at the end of the working day. They work far better than alcoholic drinks ever did, as they genuinely help me relax and they do not punish me later on.

Seana Smith

So, what do we drink when we have ditched the booze?

If I'd been writing this book even five years ago, there wouldn't have been a lot to say, but the market for low and alcohol-free drinks has changed beyond all recognition.

At one time it really was a case that the option for non-drinkers was Coke or warm orange juice. A lime and soda was as far as any bar could go. Thankfully, with the rise in numbers of people choosing not to drink as well as those people who aren't drinking due to their religion/pregnancy/breastfeeding/driving/whatever, the big producers as well as the artisan breweries have brought us a veritable array of choice.

At a recent Mindful Drinking festival in London, there were at least 35 alcohol-free beers, not to mention alcohol-free wine, alternatives to spirits and a whole host of interesting tonic waters, shrubs and kombuchas and much more. Kombuchas are a wonderful, low sugar alternative to wine. Most bars that can make a cocktail can make a mocktail and there's no need for them to be too syrupy and sweet. If you get a chance, treat yourself to a mocktail-making workshop; it's great fun and then you can impress your friends by inviting them over to sample your creations.

If you are unsure about the whole issue around the labelling of low and no alcohol drinks, 0.5 per cent ABV is classed as alcohol-free – 0.5 per cent is roughly the same amount of alcohol as there would be in a banana. If you want to avoid any trace whatsoever, opt for something that is labelled 0 per cent.

Of course, some people who ditch the booze don't want even to be reminded of it, so they don't want alcohol-free beer, wine or spirits. If that's the case for you, you still have masses of choice: there are now some amazing artisan juices and aromatic tonics.

You can make a simple refreshing drink by placing slices of cucumber in a large bowl of water with fresh mint, slices of lemon and ice. Leave it for a few hours in the fridge, then strain off the liquid and add sparkling water.

There really is no excuse to feel left out.

I've had the odd wobble. For example, I saw a couple of neighbours out walking and they shouted to me: 'We are heading to the garden for a well-deserved glass of rosé!' For a split second I felt jealous and wanted a glass…. So into the house I stomped, opened my fridge and poured a glass of alcohol-free rosé, plonked myself down in the garden and within five minutes, I'd realised I was just a bit lonely. My inner toddler wanted a play date! I wanted to sit with my girlfriends on a sunny day and laugh and have a drink… the contents of the glass was irrelevant! It was a really great moment to realise this.

Charlotte Selmon

Often when it comes to drinking, it's the ritual involved that we desire. For most of us, it wasn't a case of downing copious amounts of warm wine in a plastic cup, it was the pop of the cork, the nice glass, the ice and slice of lemon in the glass. It's super easy to recreate that ritual and concoct a fantastic drink which looks amazing. Always have some lime and lemons, add a sprig of rosemary or a mint leaf, drop a couple of frozen berries into a glass of tonic, or a twist of orange; you can have all the glamour without the booze.

So, keep the ritual, change the drink! At first, being sober and social can seem impossible, people fear their days of having fun are over. In fact, most people find the opposite is true. If people are boring, they really are, and when you were drinking, the alcohol made you more tolerant. How much better to spend your time with people you actually want to be with.

Have fun! And yes, you can dance sober, you really can!

Chapter 12
SETTING GOALS. JOURNALING AND VISION BOARDS

I n the early days and weeks of my sobriety I went to bed early many nights and wrote in my journal. I cannot recommend highly enough how therapeutic it can be to write down everything you are feeling. Clare Pooley, author of *The Sober Diaries*, started blogging not because she expected anyone to read it but because she just wanted to get it out. Keeping the thoughts and fears inside doesn't help. Getting it down on paper or screen definitely does.

You may be aware of Julia Cameron's bestselling book *The Artist's Way*. It was a ground-breaking book for its time and it's still popular. Julia believes that the bedrock of creativity is what she calls morning pages. First thing in the morning you write at least three pages of words – yes, on paper and by hand, which helps the cognitive brain (see Chapter 18 for more details). This is not your best poetry or thoughts, just a stream of stuff that comes to mind. I looked back at some of my journals from the early days and it was eye-opening to see how I was feeling, but without doubt getting that all out was therapeutic. This is not for anyone else to read – and you may or may not go back and read these journals.

Trust me, follow this guidance and you will begin to emerge from your alcohol-fuelled existence. It really is like shedding a skin; you will have more energy, and an increased sense of purpose may come along with that too. Many people find that once they have ditched the booze they find they have more time, feel more brave, and are able to actually get on with fulfilling their purpose. Often a sense of balance needs to be brought back into your life.

Alcohol takes away your spirit – literally, it steals your joy – and giving up may be the best thing you ever do. It could make you brave enough to start a business, change jobs, form a charity, write the book you've always wanted to write.

Get back in touch with what makes your heart sing, what activities you love doing and which let you lose all track of time.

> Without the constraints that alcohol inevitably brings, I found myself with a lot more time! During lockdown, I have experimented with watercolours and painted something from my close environment, usually involving a bridge. Quite metaphorical, and many sayings spring to mind: bridge the gap, burn your bridges, water under the bridge, navigate from the bridge, etc. I'm standing at the edge of a bridge in my own life, as I plan to relocate from my lovely narrowboat to the South West of England.
>
> Eloise Coyle

You'd be amazed how many people take up new hobbies once they have freed up all the time and energy they spent on drinking: people start knitting, painting, become serious exercise bunnies, bake cakes, refurbish furniture, make their own skincare, the list goes on.

When you give up the booze, what is going to be your new hobby or purpose?

My top tip for staying sober is visualisation.

If I wake up alert in the middle of the night, I visualise that I have been working away from home all week and have a long drive home. I'm so tired that I'm falling asleep at the wheel. You have to really feel the sensation. Usually the next thing I know, it's morning!

In my early days of sobriety, I often felt anxious about accepting invitations to social events. It helped to prepare by visualising the evening in minute detail, like the falling asleep at the wheel trick. I would imagine what I would be drinking, eating and wearing, who I would be talking to and how I would be feeling, framing each detail positively. This preparation takes away any ambiguity about how you will respond on the night; you already know you will ask for sparkling water instead of wine.

> Now I've turned 60, I'm even more aware of how important it is to keep adapting my mindset to remain youthful. And this has been put to the test fully during the current pandemic!
>
> Kelly Guy

Create a vision board. This is a lovely tool for allowing your subconscious mind to decide what's going to happen for you, or at least what it wants. It's easy to do. Set aside a couple of hours and turn off your phone, prepare a whole bunch of magazines, newspapers and some scissors glue and pens. In the centre of a large piece of paper or board, stick your own photo or write your name, and then allow yourself to noodle through the mags and papers, cutting out words and pictures that jump out for you. Don't analyse it too much, just see what resonates with you. Stick them in any arrangement you like on your board or paper.

You may be surprised at what you see when your vision board is complete. The result can be magical, you may spot something unexpectedly.

You may find your subconscious mind is telling you it's time to travel, to get a pet, to write a memoir. You may find you are suddenly clear about your purpose or you might just have had a fun couple of hours sticking pics of stunning holiday locations on a bit of card!

One thing is for sure: our top priority purpose should be that we are happy. I interviewed Bronnie Ware, author of *The Top Five*

Regrets of the Dying. She was a palliative care worker and heard the same regrets over and over. One of the five was: 'I wish I had let myself be happier.' So many of us have something we want to do or see or experience. We know what might make us happy, but we are fearful – scared of what others will think of others, scared of failure. We procrastinate, we promise we will do whatever it is when the kids leave home, when the summer is over… You know the saying: Tomorrow never comes.

As Bronnie says, we can choose happiness, happiness is now. That doesn't mean life will be all unicorns and rainbows and, sadly, ditching the booze can't work that kind of miracle, but we can become better at noticing these moments.

Mindfulness is a buzzword right now, but it's crucial if we want to be in the present. We spend so much of our lives thinking about the past and the future – usually for me it was berating myself for how much I'd been drinking, or planning when my next drink would be. We can train ourselves to be present.

If you have reached the end of the first 7 days or even the first 30 days of sobriety – well done!

At the end of my first 30 days, I found it useful to jot down my long list of benefits I experienced being sober. I found at least 50! What are your Top 50?

It's been great sharing some of these nuggets of inspiration with you, whatever stage you are at. You've rocked up, that's the main thing! I hope you have enjoyed working your way through this first part of the book. Hopefully, you have found enough benefits to want to stick with it. The next part of the book will help you sustain a long-lasting sober and amazing lifestyle.

Part Two

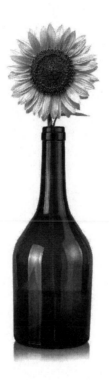

Chapter 13
STAGES OF CHANGE

ather than just focusing on one issue, it's important that we look at ourselves as a whole, our sober body (what we eat and what we drink), our sober head, our sober heart to include relationships, sex, family and parenting, and our sober soul to keep our energy flowing for ultimate health and wellbeing.

However, before we start, let's have a recap and look at our habits and behaviours with drink and the stages we go through before quitting. This will help you identify where you are in your journey.

Let me introduce you to the Stages of Change Model, also known as the Transtheoretical Model, developed in the late 1970s by James Prochaska and Carlo DiClemente who were working with smokers who wanted to quit. The model focuses on the decision-making aspects of change, looking at our habitual behaviours and how ready we are to change.

This model illustrates six stages that people typically move through, which can be helpful when focusing on ditching the booze. They are Pre-contemplation, Contemplation, Preparation, Action, Maintenance and Termination.

Pre-contemplation is the stage for many grey area drinkers, when we are unaware that we have a problem, or that our behaviour produces negative consequences. Many of us drink alcohol for years, feeling terrible, suffering hangover after hangover but, bizarrely, not making the link between the destructive behaviour and our anxiety, stress or temporary ill health.

At this stage there is no desire to change.

Contemplation is when we become aware that our behaviour may be problematic. We may start to see that our drinking is impacting on others. We start to think about reducing our drinking or think about drinking mindfully or have some alcohol-free days. The model says that at this stage people often place equal emphasis on both the negatives and the positives of making a change, so typically we might be telling ourselves we should plan a bit of a detox from drinking but also be conscious that this might affect our social life and friendships. Often we are thinking about or planning some behavioural change but don't necessarily put it into action.

Preparation is when we feel a sense of determination, and will often take some steps towards changing our behaviour, recognising that it could lead to a healthier life. This is often the time that people do an alcohol-free challenge, perhaps Dry January or Sober October.

At this stage we may realise that we aren't the only ones in this situation. When we see that there is a whole sober world of people who feel the same way and are supportive of our new healthy choices it's liberating! When I first discovered Club Soda's forum online, I felt like I had found my tribe. Community is everything!

Action is the stage where we change our behaviour and continue with this positive behaviour change, often starting to modify other behaviours in order to support these changes. We may start to realise that we have been deluded and we may discover new aspects of ourselves. Many of us start to recognise the need for self-esteem and self-care. It's also really important to be reinforcing the benefits we are feeling.

Maintenance is ongoing. It's when you have managed to sustain positive behaviour change for more than six months and have every intention going forward. In terms of sobriety, this is usually when we start to really catch sight of that better life without alcohol, and are replacing our old habits with new ones. Preparation is critically important here. We need to buy attractive alcohol drinks so that we won't 'end up' drinking alcohol because there is nothing else.

The final stage is sometimes described as **Relapse**, a common experience. Of course, the aim is not to let setbacks undermine your confidence to continue, and it's critical to ask yourself what happened before your relapse? No one just falls onto a drink, there is usually some lead-up, a thought process or some kind of emotional turbulence that went on. The relapses are, of course, what bring the learning, and we can then reaffirm our intentions and do even more preparation.

Alternatively, the final stage is **Termination**. Interestingly this wasn't added to the model until later years. This is the point when people are sure that they won't return to their original addictive behaviour and that they won't relapse. In some of the research I did, I was surprised to see that this stage is rarely reached; the majority of people stay in the Maintenance phase.

I believe, however, that a large number of us do indeed achieve this final stage. The new Sober Curious movement has made sobriety cool and something to be revered. When I asked in The Sober Club, several of my members said they were absolutely in the Termination phase and had never been happier. As one man, Alistair, said: 'After two years alcohol-free I am now most definitely a Terminator.'

If you wanted to look at the Stages of Change model from a less academic perspective, I'd say that we could bring in some qualities such as Awareness, Gratitude, Perspective and Forgiveness. Addiction and methods of help associated with it have always been quite medical and clinical in their approach, but the reality is most of us don't need clinical or medical intervention, we need connection, we need self-care and self-loving, we need to come back to who we really are, find our joy and our purpose.

Chapter 14
SOBER HEALTHY LIVING

When I take on a new client who is struggling to ditch the booze, I always ask them about their diet. Invariably they say: 'I eat really well, I eat a healthy diet', but when we start to really dig deep, it becomes apparent that it may not be healthy enough to support this roller coaster moment when blood sugar levels are all over the place and brain chemistry is out of balance.

The first thing to realise is that this isn't the time to be going on a restrictive diet. It's very common for people to have weight loss as one of their reasons for wanting to stop drinking, but your focus has to be getting properly free from the booze first. I felt very disappointed when I didn't lose weight after a few weeks of not drinking. Fortunately, I had started to see the other benefits and realise that my preferred weight, when it finally came, would be worth waiting for. Rather than a 'crash diet, quick fix, drop the pounds and pile them back on again', what happened to me was this; over time I started to love myself a bit more, I was kinder to my body and the weight that I needed to lose dropped off, almost without me noticing. Sometimes people do shed some weight in the first month, especially if they have a lot to lose, but ditching alcohol is not a magic bullet for getting slim. And there are, I'm sorry to have to tell you, cases where people put weight on before they lose it, because they turn to food instead of booze!

I worked with a client who was caught in both a food and alcohol trap: she knew it was time to ditch the booze, but she also hated her body. She weighed herself every single day, skipped meals or tried to lose weight by eating very little, and then wondered why her moods were so erratic and she felt so miserable. I convinced her to put the scales away for at least a month and focus on getting great nutrients into her body. It was incredibly hard for her at first – for her, the scales were a way to berate herself further – but I managed to inspire her to start writing her thoughts in a journal, listening to meditative visualisations and, importantly, eating three times a day, real food. The transformation was miraculous: by the time she was six weeks sober, she had lost a stone in weight (without trying), her moods had regulated, and she felt a renewed energy and enthusiasm. She was ready to kick-start the next phase of her life.

The reality is that good nutrition is the key to success in quitting alcohol. Remember the saying: 'Let food be thy medicine and medicine be thy food'. It's easy to forget the healing power of food, When our mood is low, there is much that good food can provide to help bring us back to balance.

Julia Ross is the author of the bestselling books *The Diet Cure*, *The Mood Cure* and *The Craving Cure*, and she is a pioneer in the use of nutritional therapies that successfully stop addictions and problems with mood. At her treatment centres, she has worked with many people who succeeded in curing their addictions – but only, she believes, because their diet was revolutionised. When I interviewed her for the Alcohol Free Life podcast, she told me about the first patients who came through the door. These were crack cocaine addicts, and despite giving them all the usual treatments and therapeutic sessions, all had relapsed within 24 hours of leaving the centre. She and her team decided to dig a little deeper, looking at how the brain and addictions are linked. She found that the failure of the programme wasn't to do with the emotional and spiritual treatment, though that was hugely beneficial. The core of addiction occurs in the five pleasure centres of the brain, and she found that when people were given the specific nutrients that fed the brain chemistry, their cravings would turn off and brain function became normalised. She and her team started to use nutrients to help people to feel comfort without the alcohol and drugs.

Most of us say we are looking to improve our diet, but often end up with a cross addiction, turning to other drugs, or to sugar and starch. The last thing any of us need is a food addiction to follow on from an addiction to alcohol, but it is very common.

In 'recovery' – and let's be clear, that's what it is, we are recovering after years of drinking – it's important, at least for the first 30 days, to eat three meals a day, and snacks if you need them. It's also important to include protein with every meal. Julia believes that should be specifically animal protein; she says we are carnivores and do need animal protein. This won't sit well with you if you are a vegetarian or vegan, so I suggest you really look at the protein you are eating and avoid those highly processed products marketed as vegan.

Whatever your dietary preferences, think in terms of whole foods. You can't go wrong.

Don't be afraid of carbohydrates. Healthy carbs such as fruit, beans, and complex carbs are good! Try whole grains such as millet, quinoa, amaranth and brown rice.

Omega-3s are important too. We need good amounts of EPA and DHA, so good-quality fish oils are best or blue green algae. In addition we need a balance of other omegas, from good extra virgin olive oil, coconut oil, avocado and flax seeds.

If you can add some superfoods to your diet, even better. Try sprouted seeds and beans, sauerkraut and kefir.

Protein is so important in the early stages, but you may not always want to be hitting the steak and eggs, so remember that you can get fabulous protein in the form of sprouted grains, which are, of course, more digestible than regular grains. Sprouted seeds, beans and grains are power-packed superfoods. They are full of nutrients, including antioxidants, live enzymes and vitamins and minerals. We all remember growing mustard and cress on a piece of blotting paper; sprouting seeds and beans is just as easy. You can buy special sprouting jars or trays, or just soak them for a while, then rinse and put them in some fresh water in a germinator jar. You can also use a small sieve. Mung beans or alfalfa are easy to start with; they will sprout in 3 to 6 days. Leave them to drain in a cool dark place, rinse morning and night and watch their little tails sprout! They are fantastic for adding to salads, sandwiches, smoothies and soups.

While we often set out with good intentions to eat well during the first 30 days or so, it's usually the sugar cravings that catch us out. You know I am going to tell you to avoid sugar, or at least the processed stuff. Try substitutes such as raw organic coconut nectar (which looks and tastes like brown sugar) or stevia (a plant-based sugar alternative) to sweeten. For a treat, pop a date of fig or even a few grapes in the freezer for a short while – it hits the spot!

Vegans

If you are vegan, you will obviously need to pay attention to proportions of different food groups.

You will need calcium, so go for calcium-rich plants such as seeds, dark green leafy vegetables, tofu, and plant milks which are fortified. Iodine is important and to get a good supply eat algae-based foods or spirulina capsules. Iron deficiency can be a problem for vegans, so to get enough iron eat red lentils, kidney beans, tofu and sesame. Or try the gentle and easily absorbed liquid iron.

As protein is recommended with every meal in the early weeks, prep ahead with good pulses and cereals, and soya proteins such as tofu, tempeh and nuts and seeds.

Whole grains are essential too. In addition to rice and millet, try the more unusual grains such as quinoa and amaranth, which contain good B vitamins and minerals such as iron, zinc and magnesium.

Above all when it comes to food, don't deprive yourself. Focus on what you can add in rather than what you can't have.

How do we boost our mood with food?

We've mentioned those brain chemical imbalances which affect many of us, and it's worth remembering that certain foods can help boost these important neurotransmitters. Unlike medication or even supplements (especially in the wrong quantity), natural foods won't do you any harm at all, so it's worth planning meals to include foods that boost your brain chemistry.

Serotonin is a wonderful, mood-boosting chemical, the 'feel good' chemical that makes us feel happier, enhances wellbeing, brings calm and can help with sleep. It can also help us to regulate our cravings and our hunger. If we are lacking in serotonin, we may feel irritable, panicky and experience stress and discomfort, and it's likely we will turn to food and sugary snacks for comfort. We look for something else to provide the feelings we want. Humans are pleasure seekers, so it's no surprise that so many of us turn to substances that enhance those feelings of pleasure; alcohol or recreational drugs appear to lift us, at least temporarily. They mimic the increase of serotonin, which is why we have that feeling of relief as we have the first sip of alcohol, but of course it will all come crashing down in due course. Ironically, alcohol, as well as caffeine and artificial sweeteners, lower serotonin levels, so it's not surprising that many of us are low in this important chemical.

Fortunately, the right foods will boost our serotonin levels and 'happy vibes'. One of the best essential amino acids is tryptophan, which helps to produce serotonin in the body. Foods that contain this amino acid include:

- salmon, which also includes high levels of Omega-3 fatty acids and Vitamin D
- turkey and poultry. Turkey is thought to be especially good to help with sleep
- eggs, which offer complete protein. Opt for free range and organic
- milk and cheese, which are also good sources of also calcium
- organic natural yoghurt
- soybean tofu
- avocados, which are also a wonderful source of protein and fat
- nuts and seeds, which are great for snacking or for using to make breads or crackers.

Other serotonin-boosting foods

You'll be glad to know that dark chocolate is also fabulous for boosting serotonin levels, as is pineapple, which also contains bromelain which is great for its anti-inflammatory properties. It's important to have Vitamin D rich foods too, and oils, there is more on Vitamin D later.

Dopamine is closely linked to serotonin, as it's also a mood booster, a 'happy hormone'.

When we opt for alcohol, sugary snacks and 'comfort foods', what we are doing is increasing our dopamine – but that's not a good thing! Alcohol does give us a dopamine hit, but at what cost? It's highly addictive, so we usually crave more, and the cycle continues. As we increase our intake of fatty sugary foods, they tend to increase our appetite, so we crave even more.

When our dopamine levels are out of whack, we can feel low, and lacking in motivation and enthusiasm. It can affect our memory and we may feel we have a lowered attention span. We can feel hungry and crave sugary snacks, and sleep is often impaired.

As with serotonin, we can help regulate levels of dopamine by eating proteins. Tyrosine is an amino acid that helps and can be made from phenylalanine. Let's not get too stressed about the names; the good news is these amino acids are found in the foods we've already recommended for boosting serotonin, and also in beef and legumes. Probiotics can help too, so think about sauerkraut, kimchi and kefir. Nuts, especially almonds and walnuts are good, and yet again dark chocolate is beneficial! Some studies also recommend eating velvet beans, or *Mucuna pruriens*, natural sources of L-dopa. Lentils and pulses are also great.

Another really important neurotransmitter to consider is one I knew nothing about until I worked with a nutritionist after ditching the booze: GABA – technical name gamma-Aminobutyric acid – is super important because it helps you feel relaxed and to 'chill out'.

GABA is our brain's way of putting on the brakes, slowing us up and allowing us to sleep, and regulate our mood. It can be essential for those with insomnia, and many former drinkers find themselves deficient in GABA and unable to sleep, slow down or focus.

To boost GABA, try the foods already recommended (including lentils, sprouted grains, eggs and fish), but you may want also to consider wild game, spinach, sprouted grains, oats, oranges and potatoes. Other foods high in GABA include aduki and soy beans, buckwheat, peas, mushrooms and, interestingly, white tea.

Fats

Over the years fat has had a bad rap, but don't be afraid of fats! Don't make the mistake of opting for 'low fat'. Just as 'low sugar' often equals unhealthy, because it often contains artificial sweeteners, anything claiming to be low fat is best avoided, as it usually contains sugar or other additives and synthetics. The truth is, fat isn't the baddy. We need decent amounts of omega 3, so eat organic free range eggs, avocados and oily fish. Don't forget oils, such as avocado oil and coconut oil, which is brilliant for cooking as it doesn't degrade at high temperatures. You can now get coconut butter, which is great for cooking too, and doesn't actually smell of coconut! Extra virgin olive oil is good too, and of course nut butters are great, to spread on toast or add to smoothies. See the section on juices and smoothies, page 92.

Healthy food, healthy weight

I am not a fan of calorie-counting, restrictive diets, because I don't believe they work. I am also not a fan of replacement shakes or any 'lose weight fast' approaches, though I do believe a good juice detox can kickstart the process. What really works, according to Janet Thomson, author of *The Placebo Diet*, is mindset. Janet says:

> Replacing alcohol with extra food is just like scratching the same itch with a different stick, and can itself lead to a different set of problems, so you need a really firm 'Why' you want to make the changes. A good exercise is to write down all the reasons you want to lose weight and then take a good look at the list. If there are things on there that you have said over and over, then screw it up and start again. It means you haven't got a strong enough 'Why?' because if you have been repeating those reasons and not changed, there's not enough power in them.
>
> Ask yourself 'What is the best thing that will happen when I have lost the weight?'

Then ask yourself the question this way: 'What is the worst thing that will happen if I do not lose the weight?'

With that information in your mind try this technique.

Close your eyes and remember the story of *A Christmas Carol*, where Scrooge is taken into the future and shown what will happen if he doesn't change. He feels such pain, not just for himself but for the effect his actions have on others, that he has an immediate 180° shift in his mindset. Imagine you can travel into the future and honestly look at how it will pan out if you keep old habits, drinking, eating the wrong food, and in fact anything that erodes your health. Spend a long time going into the future and honestly allow yourself to acknowledge that these behaviours cause you not just physical but also emotional pain.

If you do this properly to the point where it's truly painful to watch, and you then repeat the exercise several times (especially just before going to sleep), your unconscious mind will start to make changes for you.

As humans we are programmed to avoid pain, but sometimes we have to redefine our pain. In this case the pain caused by continuing to drink or overeat. If you keep telling yourself: 'I deserve this treat' and reaching for a cream cake, then you are not being honest. A cream cake is not a treat, it's an assault on your blood sugar.

When you have a mindset based on health and vitality, you don't need to count calories. In *The Placebo Diet* the motto is: '*Love the foods that love you back*'. In other words, no matter how much you love biscuits, crisps, cakes, they don't love you. Your body is your home, so don't let anything in that will destroy it, no matter how good it looks or tastes.

Janet Thomson, *The Placebo Diet*

Anti-ageing diet

I believe we get younger when we stop drinking! Obviously, we also need to support our sobriety with good nutrition and hydration. And as we age, good nutrition is even more important. I spend a good proportion of my time reminding people of the old saying: 'You are what you eat.' You are also what you put on your skin. I loved interviewing Star Khechara recently, an author and creator of The Facelift Diet – worth it for the name alone, right?

Stars tells us, 'Eat the rejuvenation rainbow!' In her previous career as a skincare product formulator, she noticed how many foods were popular ingredients in cosmetics and used to wonder why we are relying on tiny percentages of these foods in a moisturiser instead of eating these skin-foods in abundance in our diets. That was the start of her 10-year study into nutrition, skin and ageing.

One of the most exciting discoveries along the way is learning that beauty is more than skin deep. In fact, how we look on the outside is a direct reflection of how healthy and vibrant we are on the inside. Star says:

There are three universal truths about anti-ageing:

1. There are no neutral foods. Every bite is either rejuvenating and beautifying your body or ageing it.
2. 99.9% of the anti-ageing compounds and nutrients are in plant foods.
3. Most of those compounds are found in colourful fruits and vegetables – especially fruit, which I call the Number 1 anti-ageing food.

Eating the rainbow is a cute concept but it has a solid scientific basis: the pigments in plants which give the food its colour are also vitamins and phytochemicals that rejuvenate us and make us vibrantly healthy.

Red foods – such as red onion, strawberries, tomatoes, raspberries, red pepper and watermelon – contain compounds such as lycopene and ellagic acid, which protect the skin from UV damage.

Yellow/orange foods – such as mango, pineapple, oranges, yellow peppers, sweet potato and carrots – contain carotenoids that are powerful antioxidants which buffer the effects of 'cellular rusting' (oxidation) and also protect the skin from sun damage.

Green foods – such as spinach, avocado, cucumber and lettuce – are rich in anti-ageing chlorophyll and minerals that are essential for the healthy functioning of the skin.

Blue / purple foods – such as blueberries, blackberries, plums, purple sweet potato and purple carrots – contain the potent rejuvenating compound anthocyanin.

Eating two servings a day from each colour category will give you the full profile of anti-aging, skin-beautifying compounds your body needs.

Eat the 'rejuvenation rainbow' to slow down the ageing process all the way down to the cellular level. With so much juicy plant food in your diet, you'll naturally see your body shed excess weight as well as give you a huge increase in energy.

Star also recommends this breakfast smoothie:

Purple Rain

300 g blackberries (these can be frozen, for a cold thick smoothie)
350 g almond yoghurt
2 organic bananas
finely grated zest of 1 organic lemon
pinch of Himalayan pink salt
2–4 tsp acai powder
300–400 ml organic almond milk

Blend everything together. Pro tip: Sieve out the blackberry seeds to make it extra smooth.

Split into 2 servings – enjoy one now and bottle one to store in the fridge.

This smoothie is a powerhouse:

Blackberries and acai are rich in the antioxidant compounds anthocyanins. Not only are anthocyanins known to protect against UV damage and to be powerful antioxidants that prevent the 'cellular rusting' that instigates ageing but preliminary studies are also showing that anthocyanins can increase the levels of collagen, elastin and hyaluronic acid in skin. Eat your purple foods for youthful skin – even after menopause.

The fruit also offers Vitamin C, a potent antioxidant which scavenges Reactive Oxygen Species (ROS) – the bad guys that age skin and cause 'cellular rusting' – and protects against UV skin damage. Vitamin C is also essential for collagen production within the dermis.

Limonene, found in the essential oil in citrus peel, is known to be protective against skin cancer.

Manganese, found in nuts and the banana, is a mineral that is a known co-factor in the synthesis of collagen.

Star Khechara, Creator of The Facelift Diet® and founder of
Academy of Beauty Nutrition

I also asked Dr Hannah Short to talk us through some lifestyle tips, especially for women heading to the menopause. In addition to advising we stay hydrated and keep cool, she suggests that we follow a plant-based, whole food diet: 'Women who follow a plant-based diet have a lower risk of heart disease and cancer. Recent evidence suggests that they may also suffer fewer menopausal symptoms. Think "right carbs, good fats" not "low carb, high fat" or "no fat": complex carbohydrates (e.g. root vegetables, beans, oats, wholegrains) and plant-based fats (e.g. nuts, seeds, avocado, good quality olive oil) are essential for good hormonal health.'

Dr Hannah talks sense around food: 'Eat the rainbow,' she says, '*and* the alphabet: fill your plate with a wide variety of brightly coloured fruit and veg. Aim to include at least 10 different types of vegetable in your meals each week. Diversity is key to a healthy gut microbiome and good hormonal and emotional health.'

Hannah also recommends including minimally processed soya foods in your diet, including edamame beans, tofu, tempeh, miso

– helpful for menopausal symptoms, heart and breast health. She adds that we should flavour our food with all manner of herbs and spices.

She advises minimising refined/processed carbohydrates and junk food (e.g. refined sugar, white bread, baked goods, takeaways).

Finally, she suggests we aim to eat all meals within a 12-hour window e.g. between 7 a.m. and 7 p.m. Apparently this helps with weight maintenance and hormonal balance.

Juices and smoothies

Many a new health and fitness regime can be kick-started by juicing. I've been writing about juicing for a long time now, which has been a big part of my life since I first experienced a Juice Detox retreat. It revolutionised my life – sounds dramatic, but it's true! Jason Vale is the Juice Master who inspired me. His books are fantastic (and he wrote *Kick the Drink ... Easily!*) and if you can treat yourself to one of the juice detox retreats you won't be disappointed.

Over the years, having a fresh juice most days became so much part of my life that I had almost forgotten how important it really is – to boost immunity, and to boost wellbeing in early recovery. We all go through phases when we forget what works for us, and it took me a few weeks when I first ditched the booze to get back into the habit of drinking juices daily, especially to lift my mood and boost my energy levels.

If you are completely new to juicing, don't skip this section. Don't be confused into thinking that I am talking about 'carton juice', either. I'm referring to freshly extracted juice and smoothies that get the important nutrients straight to the cells. I must confess I first went on the detox to lose weight, and I certainly did. Losing quite a few pounds in the first week and then continuing to steadily lose weight over about a year, inspired me to really look at the importance of food with a high water content and the absolute necessity for fresh fruit and veg. Forget '5 a day'. Most of us know it should be closer to 10 or 15 portions!

It helped me be a much better parent too; I could sneak all manner of dark green leafy veg, even beetroot, into a glass if it was blended with pineapple juice! Finally, the kids were getting some decent stuff!

Juicing has had a somewhat bad rap recently. Some people claim that we wouldn't naturally consume so much fruit and veg in liquid form and that what we really need to consume is the fibre. Both points are true, but I haven't ever advocated drinking the juice of three oranges daily. I choose to have a very small amount of fruit with decent amounts of dark green leafy veg, and you can't really go wrong with that. Who doesn't benefit from a handful of cruciferous veg, with lemon, ginger, cucumber and celery?

With the best will in the world, the reality is that days go by if we are busy and we have 'forgotten' to eat lots of veg. Drinking it instead can be a quick fix, and it's an amazing energy booster, you almost feel 'plugged in'.

The fibre argument is important, but we can eat soft fruits and yet more veg to get our fibre that way. Or try what I have come to enjoy – one part fresh juice, one part smoothie.

Buying a juicer

It could well be that you have a juicer stashed at the back of your cupboard. If not, have a look at the wide range on offer, and choose the one that you will use daily! The more expensive ones are the masticating juicers that literally squeeze the juice from the fruit and veg; they yield lots of juice and are great, especially for those who are juicing to heal from an illness, as they keep all the nutrients intact.

The downside is that they are more expensive, can be fiddly to put together and to clean, and they usually have a very small chute, so you need to chop the veg into small pieces – but there is no denying the quality.

The other type of juicer is the centrifugal, which whizzes the fruit and veg round at high speed to extract the juice. (Absolute raw food 'purists' might say you are degrading the fruit and veg with the high speed which equates to heat.) These usually have a wide chute, so it's simple to just pop a whole small apple in and the whole setup and cleaning process is much quicker.

When I first heard about making a fresh juice, I wasn't sure about the actual technique. What I learnt from Jason was that the easiest way, especially if you have a relatively simply centrifugal juicer, is to have all the ingredients ready and then make a kind of 'produce sandwich' to fit into the juicer. For example, you can place one small apple into the chute, followed by a chunk of apple and fresh ginger, and then another small apple, and *then* press the On button. In other words, push a whole bunch of fruit and veg through the machine at once, it makes it much quicker.

Once you have your jug of juice, clean the juicer straight away; it makes it so much easier and then you have your juice to look forward to! Don't forget you can use some of the fresh pulp left behind as a great antioxidant, live enzyme face mask. (If you've made a green juice, be careful not to open the door to anyone!)

Most juices need a sweet–ish base such as apple, carrot, pineapple or beetroot. There is usually no need to peel the fruit and veg, especially if it's organic, which lets you hang on to the nutrients on the skin. Obviously, oranges do need to be peeled, as do avocados and bananas.

Once you have your base of apple, carrot, pineapple or beets, it's simple to concoct juices. Just use a small amount of the base, then add chunks and handfuls of whatever else you want to add. Start simply: make fresh orange juice, just to see for yourself the difference between the stuff you buy in cartons. Juice Pink Lady or Gala apples with a chunk of lemon and ginger and serve over ice – perfect!

Other favourites include carrot with ginger and apple, and beetroot and pineapple (kids love that one). You can juice watermelon, gala melon, and also herbs. Truth is, you can juice anything (well, except onions and potatoes!).

To get you started, try the 7-Day Juice Cleanse, and check out any of Jason Vale's books, especially *7lbs in 7 Days Super Juice Diet*. It's a great way to kick-start weight loss, though I highly recommend that you don't try this in the first 30 days.

Smoothies

Ideally, you'd have a juicer and a blender, but if you can only get one, get yourself a high speed blender. The really cheap ones can't cope with veg, so it's worth spending a bit more.

Throw in all the greens you'd rather not eat in high quantities – chunks of broccoli, courgette, even Brussel sprouts, spinach, kale, any combination you like. You will need something like apple juice to sweeten.

Obviously many people want to make smoothies and hang on to all the fibre, an excellent way to get a whole host of minerals and nutrients straight in! But don't be confused into thinking that a smoothie has to mean bananas and berries; the best way is to make veggie smoothies. Make it easy by juicing first, and then adding soft ingredients.

Here's a good one to kick off with!

The Green Smoothie

> 2 apples or 2 chunks of pineapple as a base
> chunk of broccoli stalk
> small handful spinach
> 5 cm piece of cucumber
> 2 cm bit of celery or fennel

You can replace ingredients with whatever you have – a couple of Brussels sprouts, some courgette, green pepper, pretty much anything can be juiced (apart from onions and leeks). Each veg has different health-giving properties.

You can drink this as it is, or you can go a step further and add it to your blender.

Once juiced, add to a blender with a handful of sprouted seeds, a chunk of avocado and any other additions you fancy, such as a tablespoon of Udo's Choice or flax oil. Or you may want to add yoghurt and avocado, to your smoothie to make it a meal; neither is fattening, these help to regulate the appetite so you don't crave fatty foods. You can add berries (blueberries are great) and a good quality protein powder, though choose an organic whey protein powder with no artificial sweeteners.

You can also add ice cubes.

Whizz all the ingredients up together and serve. This makes a fantastic healthy breakfast which will keep you going for a good few hours.

The juice shot challenge

If you are tempted to drink alcohol, and the wine witch is calling, I encourage you to have The Green Smoothie. No one can stomach a glass of alcohol after that!

If you can't face a litre of green juice, having a shot (a small intense version) is a great way of getting really strong nutrient dense stuff in, and there's not much to drink!

If you want to make sure you are getting the kick each day, why not try the 7 Day Juice Shot Challenge.

For shot recipes or for the full 7 day Juice Shot Challenge, go to happyhealthysober.com.

Here's one of my favourites to get you started.

The Fresh Ginger Shot

4–5 cm piece of fresh ginger
½ apple (skin on)
Chunk of lemon (peeled)
a pinch of cayenne pepper

Juice or blend together.

Hardcore? Juice just the ginger (whooah!!). It's good to have a freshly squeezed orange juice chaser ready.

Feel a cold coming on? This is incredibly antibacterial and immune boosting; you can increase the ingredients, add some lemon and simmer gently on the hob. Drink warm.

Ginger

A word about fresh ginger: amazing! It's well known for its anti-nausea benefits, though we no longer need the hangover cure, right? But it's also great for inflammatory pain and early onset cold symptoms. If your only experience of ginger in the past has been a ginger biscuit or a bit of powder added to cakes, you are in for such a treat! Don't forget to add it to stir-fries and curries too.

Garlic

Garlic can be a bit too much to eat raw, but does work in juices or smoothies. It's definitely worth it if you are feeling a cold coming on. Garlic also lowers blood cholesterol levels and is, again, anti-inflammatory.

Sugar

Try to avoid sugar – or, at least, the processed stuff. Look to use raw organic coconut nectar, which looks and tastes like brown sugar, or stevia, a plant-based sugar alternative.

In *Diet and Fitness Explained*, William Porter reminds us that when sugar enters the bloodstream the body releases insulin to remove it from the bloodstream so that the organs, muscles and cells can absorb and use it. The difference between natural sugar and refined sugar is that the refined sugar enters the blood stream far faster than natural sugar. This huge surge in blood sugar causes the body to release a surge of insulin to regulate the blood sugar. The blood sugar is then very quickly removed, which leaves too little blood sugar, which in turn causes you to feel drained and tired and in need of another hit of sugar. He calls this the sugar crash.

He adds that artificial sweeteners do not solve the problem. In fact, they cause other issues. Your brain triggers the release of insulin not only when it senses that your blood sugar is rising; it also starts the process as soon as it senses sugar entering your system. It does this through taste. Eating something that tastes sweet can kick off the release of insulin. This is the problem with artificial sweeteners; they taste sweet but contain no sugar, natural or otherwise, so consuming them can cause a similar crash to consuming refined sugar.

Porter points out that if you continually confuse your body in this way, it takes steps to counter the regularly high levels of insulin and you eventually become immune to the insulin and/or do not produce enough of it. This is what we know as Type 2 diabetes.

Detox

I'm sure you have heard yourself say: 'I'm going to do Dry January or Sober October – but I need to detox from unhealthy food too!'

It's a great idea in theory, but it rarely works. This is because we are trying to take on too much at once, and usually the change isn't sustainable. As I have already mentioned, in my opinion, ditching the booze, even if initially you are doing it as a 30-day challenge, should be your Number 1 priority!

A much more measured approach to detoxification is to think of the holistic picture. Really look at what needs to be eliminated and, importantly, what needs to be added in its place.

My go-to when it comes to detox is a boutique detox centre in the Cotswolds, The Milestone Detox. The founder is Helena Cavan and she is *so* knowledgeable about mind, body and spirit. She has this to say about detoxing:

> Better out than in! The word *detox* nowadays is more associated with health and wellbeing than the old-fashioned idea of a rehab clinic. *Detox* to me summarises a process of 'getting the bad stuff out and getting the good stuff in'.
>
> There is no such thing as a one-way detox because life is an exchange: inhalation, exhalation; contraction, expansion. When you decide to stop or lessen putting toxic stuff into your body, you consequentially choose to put in the life-giving stuff. Nobody lives in a vacuum and you'll always have to put *something* in!
>
> If you shift your lifestyle by only a small amount each month, say 8%, you will see a significant change over a year. 8% is such a small number; it might be that you start by

swapping your toxic washroom products for organic things. Next, you might decide to trade your caffeine drinks for decafs. The following month, perhaps you'll take a look at your household cleaners, and laundry soap. Begin with the easy things and gradually build integrity with yourself before tackling the more challenging things – like giving up/lessening sugar.

It's natural to detoxify, we each do it daily – our many detoxifying-specific organs and systems detoxify without our command. Internal organs such as the liver, gall bladder and gut process a lot of substances every day, filtering and using, recycling and rubbishing. External organs and processes, such as our skin and breathing, take good stuff in and expel toxins as well.

The intentional process of detoxification itself, however, when purposeful and supported, is *permission* and *a helping hand* to the body. Think of the detoxification process as putting the very best tools into the hands of artisans, so they can create and build greatness to marvel at.

When you start to detox, headaches, grumbles, pains and even a cough and sniffle are signs that the body is starting to really chuck things out. If you have been taking in a lot of toxins from alcohol or drugs, and are going cold turkey, it's best to be supported in a facility that will measure and monitor your blood chemistry so you stay safe while your body reconfigures. The Milestone Detox retreat is for anyone trying to detox, whether you have been drinking one bottle of wine a day or six cups of coffee a day. Interestingly, coffee withdrawal seems to cause more painful headaches than alcohol withdrawal. Chemically, the body is cleared of these toxins in around 7 to 10 days. It's the mindset shift/*toxic thinking elimination* that is the more challenging and enduring task, rather than the release of the toxins from the physical body!

To help the body clear the toxins, you can try some good old-fashioned things such as dry skin body brushing, drinking dandelion coffee, tongue scraping, magnesium/Epsom salt baths, oil pulling and castor oil packing – thus accelerating, empowering and activating your own systems.

Whatever you choose to do or take, do it. One thing. Then do it again. Keep doing it until it becomes the habit you don't even have to think about. Then take the next step. And day by day, you will transition to living that cleaner version of yourself, resulting in a happier and healthier you.

Water cure

Most of us know that the current recommendations for water are to drink 6 to 8 glasses a day. But do most of us drink enough? Here's what Helena has to say:

I check hundreds of people in on my detox programs, measuring the breakdown of their weight as cellular hydration, fat, muscle and bone – so that when they finish their detox retreat, and weigh in again, we know exactly what they've lost. Our protocols ensure that clients lose fat (aka toxic storage tanks), increase hydration and keep the muscles that they've got.

Over the years, I've noticed that as much as 8 out of 10 people who do a health retreat looking for increased energy, seeking clarity from mental fog and low moods, hoping to reverse a chronic condition or wanting to lose weight and slim down are dehydrated at a cellular level! When I explain that the body can't cleanse itself without sufficient clean water in the mop bucket, the light goes on and all of a sudden clients 'get' the simplest and most fundamental health concept of all: hydration is everything.

You can take the best and most expensive supplements, eat organic and avoid carbs and toxins, exercise and all the rest, but if you're not absorbing or drinking enough water, your body just can't do what it was designed to do well. Nobody would ever put a bottle of wine, a litre of Coke or a pot of tea into a mop bucket and expect a clean floor at the end, so why do we drink so much fluid that simply isn't up to the job of cleansing our bodies?

What quantity of water must we be drinking? Does one size fits all? My NHS nurse friend tells me that in hospital, 30–35 ml of fluids per kilo per day is the estimate used for supporting patients. If you weigh 60 kg, you need a minimum of 1,800 ml (1.8 l) per day, and up to 2,100 ml (2.1 l) per day. If you're used to weighing in pounds, then drinking half your body weight in fluid ounces is a good guide. So if you weigh 132 lb, you'd need to drink 66 fl oz per day. Divide that by your average large glass of 16 fl oz and your minimum is 4 × 16 fl oz glasses per day. No, it's not one size fits all.

Do your water figures. Any fluid counts as long as it doesn't contain a toxin: alcohol, sugar/artificial sweeteners or caffeine.

In her recent book, *Quench*, my American friend Gina Bria recommends we eat our 'apple a day' after drinking a tall glass of water – the fibre from the apple helps you stay moist longer. Some experts recommend a generous pinch of whole salt (grey sea salt or Himalayan) either on the tongue or into the water for every 2 litres of water we drink.

Many clients come in struggling with gut/constipation issues. Our colonic therapist helped develop a protocol of increased Omega-3 oils for each person who is less than 50% hydrated during our retreats. The results have been phenomenal with reported easier passages and cellular hydration increases of as much as 3% in as few as 5 days!

A municipal water supply system moves water into your home and wastewater out and away from it. If you think of your blood as being the water feed in to your body, then your lymphatic system is what moves your wastes away and eventually out of your body via your gut. In an environment where there is not enough water, because the majority of fluids taken in are dehydrating – containing alcohol, sugar or caffeine – the lymph becomes sluggish and the blood becomes thick. Nobody likes to sit by a quaggy polluted river, let alone to feel your own bodily rivers and streams as sluggish and inefficient. If you struggle with a foggy brain, low mood or energy, perhaps taking an inventory of your hydration habits in order to clean out your plumbing will give you some indicators of where your attention needs to go.

Helena Cavan has a free, 30-day email/text inspiration entitled *30 Blessings From Water* on: www.waterforlife.me

As to what kind of water we should be drinking, ah, that's the million-dollar question. In all the years I have been researching natural and sustainable living, and despite having written four books on holistic living, I have not found the definitive answer.

A friend of mine has his own well in the garden in deepest Cornwall. He had the water tested and it's oh so pure. For the rest of us, I think tap water has to do, but definitely after some kind of filtering. I've tried just about every filter and 'energising' gadget going, and have ended up back at reverse osmosis, which isn't the best for the planet but is better than buying and discarding thousands of plastic bottles every year.

I have finally invested in a SodaStream. Wow, I wish I had done that years ago! One quick 'psst' and voilà – sparkling water. Buy the one with glass bottles too rather than plastic. If you actually do the maths and weigh it up against the absolute cheapest fizzy water in supermarkets, it isn't cheaper once you have bought the gas canisters, but it is *so* much more convenient and kind to the planet, much less waste and, if you use your own filtered water before you 'fizz' it, probably better quality than the cheap sparkling water in the stores.

Coffee and tea

In terms of tea and coffee and conventional soft drinks, you know the drill. Caffeine is a stimulant and can mess with blood sugar levels: it's easy to switch to a 'coffee head' when you've ditched the drink. I must fess up, that's me, but unlike alcohol, I do have an off switch when it comes to coffee, so I will allow myself one decent coffee. Still, this is an individual thing and it would be irresponsible of me not to point out that caffeine comes with its own issues, not to mention calories if you develop a passion for iced lattes etc. If you drink coffee, it's probably best with a protein-based meal, and many health experts advise against drinking it after midday. If you are brewing it at home, opt for Fairtrade coffee if you can. Or try a coffee substitute such as Teecino.

Be careful of decaffeinated coffee, though, as the decaffeination process isn't ideal (it contains solvents), so if you're brewing decaf at home opt for the Swiss, water-based decaf process.

I went through a phase of drinking what I called a Maca Laca. This was made with maca root powder, which has excellent health-giving properties with raw cacao, boiling water, a drop of vanilla essence and any kind of sweetener (I used coconut nectar but you can use stevia drops).

Teas are pretty great. Of course, regular teas and green tea contain some caffeine, so beware if that's an issue for you, but Rooibos (red bush) teas are naturally caffeine free as are herbal teas. Sometimes people who stop drinking alcohol can go nuts over teas; it's not a bad addiction, so drink away – most have fabulous health benefits. Try a tisane, or make your own infusions, such as fresh mint tea.

Remember what you used to spend on alcohol (hopefully you have put that money aside in a glass jar and are watching it mount up!) and treat yourself to a proper, expensive tisane or proper loose-leaf tea complete with herbs and roots and flowers. You can, of course, brew your own infusion. One of the simplest is fresh mint tea: just pour boiling hot water over fresh mint leaves, leave to steep, then strain and serve, with a slice of lemon to taste.

Mindful drinking

The rise in low and no alcohol drinks is well received by the Mindful Drinking movement and the queen of all of this is Laura Willoughby from the online community Club Soda.

I first came across the work of Club Soda when I was around two months sober, feeling very isolated and wondering why I was the only one … I wasn't, I just needed to get connected. Club Soda run Mindful Drinking festivals and host forums and workshops. Meeting two of the co-founders, Laura and Jussi, introduced me to a whole new world where people still enjoyed socialising, but with non-alcoholic drinks.

In the first couple of weeks, when I became quite fixated on having my alcohol-free G&T or my alcohol-free fizz, I must con-fess I did wonder whether I was just swapping one addiction for another. Could I get addicted to those drinks? But Laura reminded me that they aren't addictive, any more than fruit is, so overdosing on them is highly unlikely. She said she has never met anyone who had an issue with them or who has felt that drinking alcohol-free drinks led them back to alcohol.

I asked Laura to share her story – and explain the often confusing labelling on alcohol-free drinks:

> I gave up drinking over eight years ago. I was inspired to create Club Soda because I wanted to help people take a self-guided journey to change their drinking, like I had. Since then, our courses and community have helped thousands of people cut down, take a break from drinking or quit altogether.
>
> Behaviour change science tells us that if you want to alter your habits, substituting one behaviour for another can really help. If you're doing something that is harmful to you or doesn't make you happy, you need a good substitute to put in its place. So choosing a low or no alcohol drink isn't just a good thing in its own right. If you're someone who's been wrestling with alcohol and trying to make changes, one of the easiest things you can do is to find something else to put in your glass.
>
> When you're looking for a drink, you'll want to choose something that is 0.5% ABV (alcohol by volume) or less. Labelling laws are complicated and inconsistent around the world, but in many countries, 0.5% drinks are described as alcohol-free.
>
> Alcohol occurs naturally in all sorts of foods, from brown bread to ripe bananas, and 0.5% really is just a trace. It can't get you drunk, it's not addictive and it's safe if you're pregnant or driving. There are all sorts of drinks up to 0.5% that could become a new favourite for you: beers, wines, spirits, kombuchas, shrubs, sodas, tonics and more. The amount of innovation in low and no alcohol drinks right now is frankly astonishing. Consumers in the UK and beyond are getting excited about innovative drinks that tickle their taste buds and you could join them.
>
> Experiment. Find a new favourite. And enjoy.
> Cheers!
>
> Laura Willoughby MBE, *Club Soda co-founder*

You can find over 1,000 low and no alcohol drinks on the Club Soda Guide at clubsodaguide.com

Alcohol-free drinks – where to start

There really are no rules when it comes to alcohol-free drinks. What was once a sugary kids' drink, the mocktail has now morphed into a cocktail that happens to be alcohol-free.

Camille Vidal from La Maison Wellness is a leading voice in the drinks industry and a Wellness Specialist on a mission to bring mindfulness into the glass and to show the world that tasty doesn't have to be boozy! She suggests mindful cocktail recipes and offers how-to videos on how to make a cocktail delicious – as she says, this has very little to do with the amount of alcohol in the glass! If you ever get chance to attend one of Camille's cocktail making workshops, they are excellent.

I recommend the Spritz Up – a refreshing spritz to boost positivity and the immune system. It's full of lovely ingredients such as apple cider vinegar, apple and lemon juice, honey water, liquid vitamin C and a splash of tonic or soda water.

You can find Camille's glamourous yet simple ideas for a drink in the recipes on La Maison Wellness website: www.lamaison wellness.com/recipes

Other simple ideas include a glass of sparkling water with a couple of red frozen berries dropped in; and of course we know that adding a slice of orange, lime or lemon or cucumber and fresh mint makes everything fab. You can add a tiny amount of artisan syrup such as Jeffrey's Tonics (see resources) or Nonsuch Shrubs or of course opt for one of the spirit alternatives, such as Sea Arch, Gin-esque and Seedlip.

You can buy readymade mocktails such as the artisan Sipling, and then there are unique blends such as Binary Botanical, which is known as the wine lovers' beer.

If you like your fizz, you need never fear: there are some excellent sparkling alcohol-free drinks, one of my faves is Noughty organic vegan sparkling wine and Wild Life Botanicals – Bubbles with Benefits.

One of my favourite drinks is a mocktail made using Sea Arch, a botanical alternative to gin. I asked the founder Sarah Yates to tell us about their ingredients:

> We use samphire and sea kelp, which are seaside botanicals native to the Devon coast. These add fresh coastal notes. There is also aromatic juniper for the gin lover. Blood orange for some citrus sweetness. Coriander to add another layer of complexity and cardamon spice for a lovely warm finish.
>
> We love the coast and we take our name from the dramatic Sea Arch in our hometown of Torquay, which erosion has created over time and is more beautiful because of what nature has taken away.
>
> Sea Arch, Coastal Juniper Blend has all the deliciousness of gin with none of the alcohol and it really is **more beautiful without** (our strap line). We have a beautiful marine blue bottle with our distinctive bronze Sea Arch logo reminiscent of a Devon sunset. The sand patterns on the side of the label are taken directly from an image of a Devon beach.
>
> It can be enjoyed simply as a Sea & T in a large glass with plenty of ice, a squeeze of citrus, and a premium tonic. Garnish with charred lemon and freshly picked rock samphire, if desired. www.searachdrinks.com

So, here are a couple of ways to enjoy Sea Arch.

Rhubarb Blush

- 50 ml Sea Arch – Coastal Juniper Blend
- 150 ml fresh homemade rhubarb juice
- ½ tsp cardamon syrup
- Serve chilled over ice, garnished with rhubarb ribbons.
- Top up with soda if desired.

Sea Arch Sour

- Pour 50 ml Sea Arch – Coastal Juniper Blend into a shaker.

- Add 30 ml fresh ruby grapefruit juice,
- 30 ml lemon juice,
- 15 ml sugar syrup,
- 30 ml aquafaba (vegan) or egg white.
- Shake for 10 seconds.
- Add 2 large ice cubes, then shake for a further 15 seconds.
- Strain into a glass.
- Decorate with powdered raspberries.

Seaside Sunrise

- Add 50 ml Sea Arch – Coastal Juniper Blend,
- 25 ml unsweetened cranberry juice,
- a squeeze of fresh orange.
- Top up with a light tonic.
- Serve in a large glass with plenty of ice.
- Garnish with a slice of charred blood orange.
- Finish with fresh cranberries or raspberries.

I could fill the whole book with amazing recipes, but the most fun is just to try some out. I hosted a birthday party when I was two years sober, and invited lots of people I hadn't seen in years. I decided to make it an afternoon event to avoid the alcohol issue (I know – cowardly, aren't I). We wrote, 'Mocktails, mulled wine (AF) and cupcakes' on the invitation and made it clear that people could bring their own alcohol if they wanted. It was a hit! On the stove, we had a big pan of alcohol-free mulled wine complete with orange zest and cinnamon (smelt divine), and laid out a 'drinks station' with instructions. Newbies could grab some ice, pour a shot from one of the alcohol-free spirits on offer – we had Lyre's, Sea Arch, Atopia, Ceder's and Gin-esque. Then they could add artisan tonic or soda, and finally move along to the 'pimping corner', where we had platters of fresh lemon and lime, rosemary sprigs, fresh mint, olives and, of course, some daft little umbrellas. Everyone loved it and made notes on what to buy and where from ... and then drove home.

So just experiment and enjoy becoming an alcohol-free mixologist!

The power of chocolate

I love chocolate, but then who doesn't? I recognised fairly on, though, that the stuff I had been consuming was in fact poor quality confectionery, with sweeteners, fillers, preservatives and fat.

The real deal is cacao, strong and dark and incredibly good for us. The main active ingredient is theobromine, and it also contains chromium, magnesium and manganese.

You can just drink it as you would tea or coffee. However, if you want to add milk, don't use dairy milk, which interacts with the chocolate, so use plant-based milk such as cashew or almond. Or you can just have cacao with hot water and some kind of sweetness. Some people like it with a pinch of sea salt or even chili!

Drinking chocolate is about much more than a satisfying drink. You can actually use a raw cacao drink to assist you in meditation and mindfulness.

Rebekah Shaman, author and plant-based medicine shaman, says:

> Cacao has always been considered a very powerful aphrodisiac, exotic food, and medicine, first by the Mesoamerican and South American cultures, such as the Mayans and Aztecs, and then by the Spanish conquistadors. Its Latin botanical name, *Theobroma cacao*, literally means Food of the Gods.
>
> The Mayans also called it Chocol'ha, and used the verb *chokola'j*, meaning 'to drink chocolate together', suggesting that cacao by its very nature needs to be drunk with others.
>
> However, we are not talking about industrialised commercial chocolate made by Nestlé or Kraft, that's packed full of milk, sugar and fats. In fact, the more cacao is processed, the more of its goodness disappears. We are talking about 100% cacao straight from the bean, ground down into what is known as the cacao liquor, and historically renowned for its many health benefits that support physical and psychological wellbeing.
>
> This is because cacao is packed with goodness, for our physical, mental and emotional wellbeing. It increases the blood flow to the brain, creating more mental agility, awareness and

focus. It may also delay dementias like senility and Alzheimer's, increase skin resistance to UV radiation/sunburn, keep skin smooth and elastic, slow down tooth decay, and remove heavy metals from the body. It also contains potassium, phosphorus, copper, iron, zinc and magnesium, which contribute to cardiovascular health.

As well as powerful antioxidants, cacao also contains flavonoids along with a significant amount of chromium, which balances blood sugar levels and helps the body's cells resist damage by free radicals caused by toxic environments. Likewise, the flavonoids lower blood pressure, help the clotting process of blood, and improve blood flow to the brain and heart, while the theobromine and caffeine content boosts energy levels and relieve fatigue.

Its high valeric acid content triggers the release of dopamine, anandamide and the endorphin phenylethylamine, all of which are known as the 'bliss molecules', and give us the feeling of being in love. Cacao also contains the essential amino acid tryptophan, which increases production of serotonin, an important brain chemical that helps us remain positive and happy. A lack of serotonin can lead to depression, fatigue and mood swings. Evidence from clinical trials show that consuming 1½ ounces [about 40 g] of dark chocolate per day for a period of two weeks reduced stress hormones and stress-related biochemical agents in volunteers who rated themselves as highly stressed.

Cacao is a powerful plant medicine which helps us release emotional blockages that no longer serve us, find forgiveness in ourselves and others. It also enables us to dissolve stuck emotions, conditionings, patterns of behaviour and addictions that are buried deep in the unconscious.

Rebekah Shaman www.Rebekahshaman.com

A cacao ceremony

At Sobriety Rocks retreats with Jo and Dominic De Rosa, the day begins with a cacao ceremony. Jo explains what happens:

You will be passed a cup of warm cacao, which will have been made most likely from a nut milk, as animal milk inhibits the uptake of the active compound, theobromine, in the body. In around 30 minutes, the cacao increases blood flow by dilating the arteries, thus lowering blood pressure, reducing heart disease and stroke, with one study finding cardiovascular disease was cut by 37% and stroke by 29%. It balances out good and bad cholesterols, enhances your mood, has aphrodisiac properties and is even an appetite suppressant. So along with it being packed with vitamins, minerals and antioxidants, cacao also has anti-inflammatory properties, and by consuming 20 g [¾ oz] per day you can significantly reduce the build-up of plaque in your arteries.

Not all chocolate is equal, and you need to find a good source; one which still contains the goodness and, therefore, all the above benefits. It's subtle, not like recreational drugs which give you a strong hit or rush. Cacao is soft and velvety, she caresses your heart chakra, and like a rose she entices its petals open. She shows the way to more love, deepening your understanding of yourself, the world, and your place in it. You are guided by the ceremony teacher on deep journeys through your soul, going ever further into the depths of your being. It is pure bliss, and you leave the ceremony on the most beautiful and natural high, sharing the expansiveness that you feel with everyone you meet.

There is no guilt with ceremonial grade cacao; this surely is next level stuff! When you discover cacao in its true state, you realise you can have your chocolate and eat it.

The Blissful Cacao Ceremony Recipe

Per person

Ingredients

20 g ceremonial grade cacao
20 g cashew nuts
Add sweetener to taste (we use around 1–2 teaspoons of xylitol)

Flavour of your choice: 1 teaspoon of maca / lucuma / vanilla / cayenne

Method

Put all of your ingredients into your food processor and blitz at a high speed until the cashews have broken down and you're left with a smooth drink.

In a high-powered blender, friction will heat the cacao.

In a conventional blender, you may need to warm your cacao on the hob. We heat ours to around 46°C, so it is warm – but still raw and not hot enough to cook out the goodies.

If you are not using cashews and water to make cashew milk, use any nut/coconut milk. Just not animal milk, as it inhibits the uptake of the active compounds in the cacao.

Store for up to 3 days in an airtight container/bottle in the fridge

Jo and Dominic De Rosa www.blissfulinfinity.com/cacao

Maca

I mentioned earlier that one of my favourite drinks was what I called a Maca Laca. Maca has definitely become more popular; it's an adaptogen (a substance that helps the body adapt to stress) and has many other health benefits.

Dr Michael Barnish, Head of Genetics & Nutrition at REVIV Global Ltd, explains that maca was cherished by the Inca Empire and even taken by their warriors before going into battle! The root of a plant native to the high Andes of Peru, it is a cruciferous vegetable and has been used as food and medicine in Peru for as long as records exist.

In recent years, maca has been studied for its countless health benefits and is now popular around the world, labelled as a superfood! It is highly nutritious and, dependent on the colour (it can be white, red black or purple), it contains some protein and fibre, alongside essential nutrients, such as copper, iron, potassium, Vitamin B6, manganese and of vitamin C.

Maca is also packed full of flavonoids too, with antioxidant properties; it can improve the body's detoxification ability and improve its cellular communication. Studies show it improves cognitive function, reducing the risk of cardiovascular disease and the reduction of typical menopausal symptoms.

So, amazing nutritional content!

Here's a fab recipe using Maca recommended by Dr Michael Barnish:

Maca Sweet Potatoes Recipe

- 4 medium sweet potatoes, peeled and chopped
- 1 tablespoon Maca Powder
- 2 tbsp olive oil or coconut oil
- 2 tsp chipotle paste or powder
- 1 tsp smoked or sweet paprika (depending on preference)
- 1 tsp lime juice
- small handful coriander, torn, to garnish
- salt

- Preheat oven to 200ºC.
- In a bowl, combine maca, oil chipotle, paprika, salt and lime juice, then pour over the sweet potato chunks and stir well to coat.
- Spread out evenly over a baking tray and bake for 40 minutes.
- Remove from the oven and put into a serving tray.
- Garnish with coriander before serving.

Gut health

Looking after our gut health has become a trend. A few years back, no one knew what the microbiome was, but now it pops up in the health pages of most weekend newspapers.

Our gut is our second brain. Really. We know that when we are upset, we feel it in our gut first. We have 'gut instincts'. Our gut health rules just about everything else and, sadly, over the years we have managed to slowly deplete much of its inherent supplies of good bacteria through our poor lifestyle choices and environmental toxins.

The absolute queen of gut health is Shann Jones. I first came across Shann when I heard her incredible story of how she healed her son's severe eczema using goat's milk kefir. As well as being an author she is the founder of Chuckling Goat. Here's what Shann says:

Alcohol does a lot of bad things to your body. But one of the most severe – and most under-reported – things it does is to damage your gut microbiome. Your gut microbiome is the name we give to the 2 kg [4 lb] of living bacteria that live inside your gut. This natural ecosystem is so important to your overall health and well-being that it is considered to be its own 'organ'. The best way to imagine this is like a beautiful little Amazon rainforest inside you, full of gorgeous and diverse living creatures.

The problem is that, like any natural ecosystem, the one inside your gut is fragile, and can be easily damaged. What damages it? The things I like to call the Five Horsemen of the Gut Apocalypse: sugar, stress, environmental toxins, antibiotics and – you guessed it – alcohol.

Alcohol alters the important neurotransmitters produced inside your gut, including GABA, serotonin and dopamine. Messing with these critically important substances can create massive behavioral changes, including emotional behaviour, memory, sleep alterations and depressive disorders.

So, you've quit the alcohol – great first step! You've stopped doing the damage. But how do you repair the damage that has already been done?

The good news is that your gut microbiome is one of the easiest 'organs' in your body to affect using food. Rebuilding your gut health can be accomplished using a combination of **probiotics** and **prebiotics**.

Step 1 – Drink probiotic kefir

Probiotics are living beneficial bacteria that can repopulate your microbiome and restore the health of your gut. Dr Michael Mosley on his BBC2 show *Trust Me I'm a Doctor*, found that a natural fermented drink called kefir was the most effective probiotic food available on the market today.

Step 2 – Take a complete prebiotic

In addition to probiotics, it's important to take prebiotics for optimum gut health. In a nutshell, prebiotics are food for probiotics. If you imagine that a probiotic like kefir puts the 'fish back into the river' inside your gut ecosystem, then those fish need to be fed. But what do you feed the fish, to keep them alive?

Gut bugs eat fibre. Recent science reveals that there are 21 different types of fibre required by your gut bugs to keep them healthy. These fibres include exotic items like maitake mushrooms, cassava root, and tamarind powder – not things ordinarily found in the British diet.

A complete probiotic combines multiple natural sources of prebiotic fibre into an easy-to-use powder. Probiotic kefir and prebiotic powder can be blended into a gut-health smoothie, as a daily part of your inflammation-busting routine. www.chucklinggoat.co.uk

I cannot stress enough the importance of good nutrition, especially in the first few weeks and months after quitting the booze. There are different expert opinions, recipes and tips and of course a wide variety of diets that you can try. The most important thing to remember is that alcohol can strip away key nutrients, so it is likely that you will be depleted in those natural feel good chemicals. That's why focusing on a 'recovery diet' which is nutrient dense and not restrictive is so key. As with everything, there is no one size fits all programme, but if it's 'real food', and you know it's good for you, you can enjoy it!

Chapter 15
THE SOBER MIND

have said at length in the first chapters that I think it's important to educate yourself about what alcohol actually is and what it does to us emotionally. William Porter explains:

> Alcohol is a sedative, which means it inhibits or depresses nerve activity. When we drink, our brain senses that the internal delicate chemical balance has been upset and it counters the sedating effects of the alcohol. It does this in various ways which amount to it becoming increasingly sensitive so that it can function under the sedating effects of the alcohol. The alcohol then wears off, leaving the brain overly sensitised for a period before it then recalibrates and returns to normal.
>
> This period of over-sensitisation is what is known as 'hangxiety'; that period of increased anxiety that is the 'comedown' from drinking. It is alcohol withdrawal; a distinctly unpleasant feeling that we get when the initial effects of the alcohol are wearing off, and it can be relieved by another dose of alcohol. The anxiety is caused by your brain being calibrated to work under the sedating effects of the alcohol, but without the alcohol it's in disarray. When you then drink again you experience a wonderful, relaxed, comforted feeling as the anxiety caused by the previous drinking is relieved. This is the main benefit of drinking for regular drinkers; they are relieving the anxiety caused by the previous drinks. The feeling of relaxation and

comfort is, in fact, just returning temporarily to a state they would already be in had they not drunk in the first place.

Of course, the more alcohol you consume, the greater the comedown or withdrawal is. Too many spirits will leave you with the shakes, panicky, depressed and completely unable to function. One glass of wine will leave you feeling a bit out of sorts and anxious. Many people have lived and died without ever consciously identifying that increase in anxiety; still less do they see their daily drinks as just the regular relieving of the alcohol withdrawal. All they know is that a drink makes them feel comforted and relaxed.

Returning to normal when quitting alcohol is a four-stage process:

1. The alcohol needs to leave your system, which usually takes up to 24 hours.
2. There is then the overstimulation phase, where you will feel overly anxious and possibly have problems sleeping (this is usually over within 1 to 5 days).
3. If you are a regular drinker, your brain will have been overly sensitised most of the time since you started drinking. Now that it no longer needs to be in this state of constant over-stimulation, you may feel lethargic and sleep a lot (similar to if you were used to drinking a lot of caffeine and suddenly cut it out). This can last for up to 3 weeks.
4. You will need a few nights to catch up on proper, restful sleep.

When you are through this, you will feel better than you have since you started drinking. This is the great secret of sobriety!

William Porter, *Alcohol Explained* and *Alcohol Explained 2: Tools for a Stronger Society.*

Limiting beliefs

We think that we are weak, we think that there is something inherently wrong with us, that we have an addictive personality, which is why we have failed time and time again to stop drinking. If you are reading this book and are still in the early stages, I would wager that you have had or still have issues with self-esteem. Who doesn't? Most of us simply don't love ourselves enough; we don't believe that we are enough.

I'm not talking about having a big ego, being narcissistic or thinking you are better than everyone, I'm talking about that feeling of being authentic, of valuing yourself. I spent years promoting meditation, mindfulness and self-care, but if you'd asked me if I loved myself, I would have laughed and said, 'Hell, no!'

It wasn't till I ditched the booze that I was able to fully understand just how much I had been using alcohol to numb the feelings of inadequacy, of insecurity, of fear and anxiety.

Most people reading this will be aware of the theory that we are born without limiting beliefs, which are established during our formative years. It may be that a parent tells you that you are stupid, or someone calls you ugly, or worthless. It can be anything. As a rational adult, you would be able to evaluate the statements or accusations, and probably see quite quickly that they aren't true, but the child doesn't have that ability and instead stores them away as proof to be on your guard in future: you feel you mustn't speak up because your voice and opinion are not valid.

Of course, these thought processes aren't conscious, but all of these limiting beliefs are stored in your unconscious mind and they impact your every move. Each of us has our baggage, our collection of beliefs about ourselves that hold us back. Sometimes we have surpassed our own fragile hopes and managed to be successful, we have held down good jobs, appeared confident, enjoyed meaningful relationships and yet still something is holding us back.

NLP expert David Snyder describes this as *Going through life on a speedboat with a high octane fuel jet engine...but a huge anchor creating the drag.*

If we want to set ourselves up to succeed and achieve what we want, then we must try and shift those anchors and clear the limiting beliefs holding us back.

This is extremely common, by the way. When I work one to one with clients, I find that in almost every case there has been some level of childhood trauma. Children take things personally, so when something happens to a child that they perceive as 'bad', they often see it as their fault.

Dr Gabor Mate is an expert in childhood trauma and talks extensively about the ACE study, which draws attention to the impact of Adverse Childhood Experiences. What's needed according to Dr Mate is a compassionate approach to addiction, where we recognise that many of us suffered in childhood, and the root of over-drinking, over-eating, over-exercise, whatever the issue is, comes from our early childhood rather than from a genetic failing, disease or being a hopeless person.

We can't go deep into counselling and therapy here, but there's no doubt that the more you acknowledge your early suffering and the limiting beliefs that formed as a result, the more you can move forward. I always recommend counselling and therapy for those with trauma that has been buried deep for a long time. There is no doubt that when we remove alcohol from our life, we may have to face up to some of the more tricky stuff.

David Synder – hypnosis and NLP trainer says – and this is a powerful statement: *Things that hold us back often aren't our fault, but it's our responsibility to get rid of them.*

For most of us, our limiting beliefs impact every decision we make. Some people decide quite early on that they will drink alcohol because they have formed a set of beliefs by watching others around them. Perhaps they saw other teenagers looking 'cool' smoking or drinking, or perhaps they felt shy around others they were attracted to and then found that alcohol lubricated everything and made them feel confident. A belief was formed at that point: alcohol makes me feel good, confident, relaxed, and happy.

These limiting beliefs can seriously impact our decision to ditch the booze because while we know we 'ought to' and we say we 'want to' be free from alcohol, we are weighed down with thoughts of 'but I won't feel confident, attractive, I won't have fun anymore'.

The way to start working with our limiting beliefs is to notice them and then question.

It's key to remember that they are just beliefs, they aren't facts. For example, night follows day is a fact. My commonly repeated statement that I am clumsy and drop things is a belief. It's just a thought that I have on repeat. But, I can notice it, I can ask if it is always true, and then I can be 'curious' about how to reframe it.

We can work with our limiting beliefs and change them, and over time we can build up a whole new collection of memories and beliefs that support good self-esteem and feeling happy as a non-drinker.

Ask yourself what fundamental limiting beliefs you have and what you'd like to change in your life. Be your own private investigator and ask yourself: *What's really stopping me?*

You are *flawsome*. I don't know who came up with the word, but I love it.

For many of us, looking in the mirror and telling ourselves we are *awesome* is a bridge too far, but *flawsome* covers it.

Often, once you ditch the booze, you start to get clarity on what you want for your life, and things start to feel more possible. Let's look a few more therapies and techniques that can really help.

NLP

NLP stands for Neuro Linguistic Programming and it's an incredible set of tools to enable you to change behaviours, deal with limiting beliefs and feel empowered. I have picked up bit of NLP over the years and have been using it in my media training work, but it wasn't until fairly recently I decided to train as a practitioner. I chose to work with Andy Coley and Jo Wilson, award-winning NLP Trainers. I loved the course and now use the techniques with my coaching clients and, of course, in my everyday life. I have found it certainly improved my relationships with my teenagers. It seemed fitting to ask Jo and Andy to share some of their knowledge of NLP with us here.

Neuro-Linguistic Programming (NLP) evolved from the fields of psychotherapy, psychology and sociology when the founders created a series of models, philosophies and tools that enable people to understand how they uniquely process the world around them, how can they stop unhelpful behaviour patterns, change the way they respond to situations, build empowered strategies and communicate with ease. In essence, NLP is:

Neuro – the study of how your mind works, how you take in and process information and the resulting version of reality that you act and react to.

Linguistic – the verbal and nonverbal language you use to communicate with others and how other people's use of language impacts you.

Programming – Many of your habits, behaviours and reactions are learnt over time and become embedded and can often feel like they are automatic. You develop strategies and run behavioural programmes, a bit like how a computer uses a program to get certain results. NLP gives you the ability to understand and then easily change the unhelpful programs that you run, get rid of negative thoughts and learn new positive habits and strategies.

Through understanding how both the conscious and unconscious minds work and the power of our unconscious patterns that we build over time, NLP enables us to make significant and lasting change.

Your unconscious mind carries out all your automated functions such as breathing, balance, digestion, etc. It also has a blueprint for you as a healthy person and will always do what it believes is best for you. In NLP terms, we call this the positive intention. The problem is that it can hold onto that positive intention for too long or inappropriately, the result sometimes being that our behaviours become self-destructive or harmful to our health, our emotional wellbeing and the things and people that are important to us. This is particularly true about addictive behaviours.

Jo was coaching a lady (let's call her Jean) who felt that she was on a self-sabotaging cycle of behaviour. Jean had a tendency to drink wine every evening. She had a very busy and stressful career and loved to unwind at the end of the day with a large glass of wine as a reward for getting through the day (her unconscious mind's positive intention for the wine was reward and relaxation).

The problem was that the glass of wine soon became two and, before Jean knew it, she was drinking a bottle each evening. In the morning she felt groggy, hated herself for drinking too much the night before and found she was putting on weight and felt sluggish throughout the day. She knew she should stop but felt that she couldn't.

The first step was to help Jean recognise that the positive intention her unconscious mind had associated with the wine was no longer appropriate. Finding replacement ways for Jean to get the reward and relaxation she craved, that were more in-line with who she wanted to be and what she wanted to achieve in her life, was a fantastic first step which led to Jean to no longer needing even one glass of wine!

Andy was coaching a gentleman (let's call him Paul) who had been drinking heavily for a while and came from a background where booze was very much part of family life. Now in his late 50s, Paul wanted to stop the need for alcohol to be his lifeline and focus on getting healthier and fitter so he could be there for his fantastic partner and his grandchildren.

Anger and frustration were a big trigger for his drinking pattern, and so Paul and Andy worked through several NLP tools that enabled Paul to focus on creating a calming state that he could access when required. They also looked at what the positive intentions were from the old anger and frustration patterns.

A few weeks later, things had changed. Paul been sleeping fantastically and was feeling much more like his old self. He'd reduced his alcohol intake down by 90%, a glass of wine with dinner during the week instead of his old intake of 30 pints, several G&Ts and four bottles a wine a week. He felt happier and looked lighter, could breathe more easily and was looking at a future full of joy and positivity.

The reasons why people start on a self-destructive road are different. By finding what motivates you to change, you know that it's possible to take a new road and head in a different direction. First, you do need to accept that the past has been and gone. You can learn from it, reflect on it and decide, now, to do something different in the future. For it is the future that you shape with the choices you make right now.

Try this out for yourself

Let's tap into our inner guru, by learning to step away from our emotions of a situation and take some powerful advice from a more empowered version of yourself.

You might want to grab a pen/paper to make notes from this exercise.

Choose something that you would like to change or achieve in your life. Ask yourself the following questions.

1. What will happen when you do make that change or achieve that goal?

2. What will happen if you don't make that change or achieve that goal?

3. What won't happen when you do make that change or achieve that goal?

4. What has been stopping you from already changing it or achieving it?

Then imagine going back in time to a much younger you, at an age when life has not yet created too many responsibilities, when you could be playful and creative. It helps if you could try to step into this role. Perhaps sit as you would have sat, move as you used to move, be as you used to be.

Ask yourself: What would this younger you say to you about what's been stopping you? What would this younger you say was missing in your life now that needs to be present? Or is there anything present that they would suggest needs to be missing for you to move forward, now?

Is there anything else they advise?

Now imagine going forward in time. Way out into your future, to a time not long before you are about to hang up your hat on this life.

With the wisdom of age and the gift of hindsight, imagine what life would be like.

Down one road is your life when you failed to make that change or achieve the goal. You kept on going in the way you used to be. What would that older you say right now? What advice would they give about what you could have done differently, who you needed to be to have achieved what was lost? As you reflect on that path and the repercussions and ripples that happened as you got older, is there anything else that older you would tell you to do, now?

Now bring yourself back to the present day and look down the other road. Imagine and see what happened when making those changes and achieving your goals. What needed to happen for this to happen? Notice the stepping stones that take you from now into the future and what that means for the older you, now.

Finally, bring back all those learnings from the past, present and futures and notice what's different. Notice who you need to be to make those changes as you step into a future full of potential.

Andy Coley and Jo Wilson www.beyondnlptraining.com

The power of EFT (Emotional Freedom Techniques)

When I first heard about EFT, I was sceptical. I had heard that it's a process of light physical tapping on various points on the body, which is said to work because energy flows along meridians that connect to each other and to our organs resembling an electrical circuit. The idea is that when we are under stress, whether physical or emotional, the energy meridian can become blocked or shut down. An analogy would be if a battery was inserted the wrong way; the device wouldn't get its power. If a negative emotion disrupts the body's energy system, it makes sense that clearing the blockage should be possible, to let the energy flow again. When you tap on the various points, you are encouraged to speak out loud and state the problem. This will almost certainly mean that you 'voice' the negative – 'I'm craving alcohol', 'I'm hopeless at looking after myself', 'I'm so greedy and putting on weight'. This went against the grain for me, I must admit. I had done so much work around affirmations, where it's important to always state the positive, in the present tense – 'I am now healthy and loving myself', 'I am at my ideal weight' and so on.

What I learnt over time is that both have value. When it comes to those deeply ingrained limiting beliefs or issues that cause us distress, though, the reality is that unless we bring them out into the open we can't deal with them. I can't remember which wise soul said: 'You can't clean the house unless you can see the dirt!'

On my first day learning how to be an EFT practitioner, I worked with another course participant who revealed an eating disorder she'd had since childhood. She didn't enjoy food, and couldn't eat with others or in a social situation. Within a few minutes of 'tapping this out', we uncovered feelings of loneliness and looked at why her unconscious mind had made her choose to be left out' at mealtimes. After only about 30 minutes she was shocked and amazed to find that she had feelings of hunger and felt comfortable to sit with the rest of the group to eat; this was something she hadn't done in over 20 years!

This is powerful stuff, and the tools can be used for all kinds of old beliefs and issues. I now use it when I am coaching clients, not just in changing habits, and boosting their health and wellbeing, but also for confidence in going after their goals.

I trained with Peter Donn, an EFT Master trainer who runs the EFT Training Centre, offering courses and sessions online and in person in Hertfordshire, UK. I asked Peter to explain exactly what it is and how it can work with addictions.

The basis on which EFT is believed to work relates to the part of the mid-brain called the amygdala. Along with associated structures, this is where emotional memory is stored. Its function is to protect us by setting a red flag against experiences that could be dangerous to us. This happens when we experience trauma. In that moment, it records the environment of the trauma (what we see, hear, smell, etc) and associates it with the emotions and feelings we felt at the time. Then, whenever we are in the presence of those same environmental 'triggers' (or we think about them) it replays those feelings. This usually happens subconsciously. Incidentally, this effect also applies to inherited 'epigenetic' trauma.

The body does this, as it does in animals, to protect us from future danger and to give us a chance to escape the threat.

In the most part, we have those experiences when we are young and helpless, and yet – despite the response having no relevance later in our lives – we continue to get triggered on an ongoing basis. This leads to a state of repeated stress and anxiety as we move through life.

What needs to happen to get relief from this is to 'tell' the amygdala that we are safe now, and that it is OK to let that association go. This is what EFT does, and does very effectively. As you tune into your body's emotional response whilst tapping, you are sending 'you are safe' signals to the amygdala and within minutes (sometimes seconds) the body starts to relax. A 2019 fMRI study relating to food cravings confirmed that EFT had the effect of deactivating that neural response.

In fact, EFT can be used – gently – to experience complete relief from even the most severe trauma to the point where you couldn't get upset even if you tried. For this kind of deep result, you would probably need the help of properly trained professionals.

EFT has been the subject of many studies, around half of which are double blind, placebo controlled. This repeatedly shows that it is effective and that it is the tapping itself that is the key therapeutic feature.

EFT and cravings/addictions

If you stop drinking without handling the underlying drivers, there's a chance you will find yourself shifting to another way to suppress those feelings, such as overeating or smoking or keeping busy to unconsciously divert attention away from the deeper feelings.

EFT can be used in two ways to help overcome cravings and addictions.

The first is by using it on a daily basis to target both general stress, emotional discomfort and the cravings themselves. By tapping repeatedly and persistently, you are etching away in the background at the deeper drivers to the point where they may be so much reduced that your cravings disappear completely!

The second way of working involves directly addressing the deeper emotional drivers. You are likely to need help from a trained EFT practitioner who can work with EFT in a more advanced way.

However, here is the basic tapping routine that you can do for yourself.

Let's say you are feeling anxious about meeting friends who will be drinking. Focus on that issue and determine the intensity, between 0 and 10, with 10 being very bad, and ask how uncomfortable is this for me, physically or emotionally?

Then do what we call a 'set-up', where you state your issue and acknowledge acceptance.

Use one or two fingers to tap on the 'karate chop' point of one hand. That's the side of the hand midway between the nail of the little finger and the wrist, and as you tap say the phrase:

'Even though I (am anxious about meeting friends for drinks tonight) I deeply and completely love and accept myself.'

If this feels alien to you, go with it anyway!

Repeat that three times. You can vary the phrase, so it might be that the second time you do this, you say: 'Even though I am worried I will feel tempted to drink…I deeply and completely love and accept myself.'

Then you go through the basic tapping sequence, on the meridian points. Using either hand (or both), tap a few times. You can state the issue out loud if you wish as you do so ('I'm worried I might be tempted to drink'). Tap:

- on the side of the eyebrow (where it meets the bridge of the nose)
- the side of the eye (above the cheekbone)
- under the eye
- under the nose
- under the lips, on the chin
- on the collarbone
- under the armpit (for women where the bra should sit)
- top of the head

Repeat your issue in no particular order as you tap to focus on the problem and then take a deep breath, after you have tapped through the sequence a few times.

When you have completed a few rounds, test your intensity level again, and see if it has gone down. If it is under 3, amazing! If there is still work to do, repeat the process.

Bear in mind this is a simple EFT exercise, and won't always work for you doing it yourself. However, an EFT practitioner will be able to show you how. Peter Donn https://www.eft-courses.org.uk/

Havening

There are other techniques said to help with stress and anxiety. I was introduced to the Havening therapy, but it's actually a psychological therapy that is gentle and safe and great at helping with anxiety and any powerful negative emotions. It's also great for resilience and confidence. The creator of the Havening technique is Dr Ronald Ruden. The well-known author Paul McKenna is a big advocate. I remember interviewing him for *Steve Wright in the Afternoon* on Radio 2 and watching as he crossed and then stroked his arms to demonstrate how Havening worked. It didn't quite come across on radio, but it definitely made an impression on me!

Havening has been described by some as Speed EFT – for someone as time-stretched as I am, that can only be good.

Havening is a technique we can do for ourselves (or work with a practitioner). It works on the state of our brain. As already described, our amygdala is the sensor which decides if an event is safe or threatening. If it perceives a threat, and our old beliefs are already vulnerable, we may feel we have no way out. Hence we sometimes feel stuck or out of control. The Havening Touch can help to restore new patterns, removing the charged emotional response. To increase a positive emotion we can use gentle calm movements, moving our hands across our arms or across our cheeks. This creates the delta wave, similar to deep sleep, which changes the state of our brain and alters the chemical balance to increase our serotonin and decreases our stress levels, to make us feel calmer. It dissolves the pathway so that if the negative trigger occurs it's not linked to the emotional response, and the memory may no longer be traumatic, and instead be just a memory.

I met with Tam Johnson the founder of Fresh Insight Coaching. She is a life coach, NLP master practitioner and hypnotherapist, and works with people who have anxiety or stress, issues with self-esteem and confidence, even deep-rooted emotional trauma (from PTSD to sexual abuse). Conventionally this can take years to abate, and Tam has managed it in just a few sessions. She cured her own severe phobia of heights, using the Havening technique as she stood at the side of a cliff top with no side effects. After 30 minutes she was able to fully enjoy a spectacular view for the first time in 20 years!

With a very no-nonsense approach, Tam asked me to imagine myself as someone else, a different version of myself watching my own state of mind and my actions. It was enlightening to see how she guided a different perspective. As she says, 'I step into my client's shoes and see the world through their eyes to create the changes *they* need.'

We all tell ourselves stories as to how we are feeling, what is holding us back, what has been done to us, but Tam is the ultimate 'happiness catalyst' and believes it is possible to establish new patterns. Just as our computers sometimes become overloaded and go a bit weird, needing a reboot, so we sometimes need to reprogramme our thoughts and our responses. Tam taught me to pause and notice what was going on when I had certain negative thoughts and encouraged me to use a simple Havening technique as often as possible, for at least 10 minutes a day.

Tam explains how easy to do this for yourself:

'Just cross your arms and slowly stroke downwards from the shoulder to the elbow. You need to focus on the emotion, so say to yourself, 'I am confident, I am powerful' (or whatever state you want to focus on).

You can also slowly use your palms as if you are washing your hands in a slow, steady way and repeat the positive state you want to feel. You can intensify the technique by closing your eyes and visualising going up a staircase with 20 steps. Count from 1 to 20 out loud as you ascend in your imagination. When you are at the top hum a few lines of a familiar song such as 'Happy Birthday' (while still stroking your arms). Finally take a deep breath and open your eyes, look from right to left, close your eyes, inhale and exhale. Continue with the Havening arm stroking and ask yourself if the feelings of anxiousness/negativity have abated.

Havening is such a simple soothing technique it has to be worth a try. You can even lie in bed Havening. I defy you not to drop off to sleep, or do it for five minutes when you take a loo break.

Tam Johnson http://freshinsightcoaching.com/

Therapeutic treatments for the body

In addition to the techniques that help us psychologically, I believe that there are times when we just need to go for the somatic and look after our body.

When we are feeling any kind of discomfort, we tend to go off into our heads, revving up the destructive thoughts, panicking and creating all kinds of physical responses through our negative thought patterns. Another option is to just drop onto your mat.

Literally lie down and breathe, or sit with your back against a tree. Walk in nature, preferably barefoot, and come back to the body.

What is happening in the brain affects the body and vice versa. If we think about a delicious snack, we can literally find ourselves salivating; if we suddenly hear horrific news, we have an immediate discomfort in our stomach or break out into a sweat.

Psychologists call this the cybernetic loop – what happens in the body affects the brain, and it works the other way too. So when our thoughts are chaotic, when our mind is whirling and fears and thoughts are raging, we can literally encourage our body to feel calm and strong.

This is why the Power Pose works so brilliantly. When we stand with feet firmly planted into the ground, arms by our side, head up, we send a message to the brain: 'I'm OK, I'm strong.' This is such a simple way to boost our own feelings of wellbeing before any important meeting, or even just to take a moment out of a stressful situation.

If you are feeling anxious and stressed, stand up tall, look up, think of your favourite colour, perhaps go back to an image of your 'happy place' – and breathe. You can place your hand on your heart too and feel the stress melt away.

Bodywork is extremely beneficial when you are ditching the booze, and beyond. The power of touch can't be denied. I love aromatherapy, reflexology, reiki, lymphatic drainage, and Bowen therapy, to name just a few, but any and everything that makes you feel good will be beneficial. Treat yourself.

One unusual treatment that I experienced soon after ditching the booze was Trauma Release Exercise (TRE). It is sometimes re-ferred to as 'shaking meditation'. We've all seen mammals shake and tremble, especially when they have just been released from trauma (perhaps they have had to run away from another animal) and we can do the same to release our stress.

This mild 'involuntary' shaking action literally gets rid of the old energy, especially when our fight or flight impulses have been triggered. So if you have had a stressful or upsetting event – shake! It activates the parasympathetic nervous system and sends a message to the brain to allow you to calm down.

If you can be taught how to do it, even better. It's difficult to describe, but it worked on my energy system and I felt quite different after leaving Nadia Smith's woodland therapy room.

Nadia Smith is an holistic practitioner and author of *True To My Roots* and founder of True To Our Roots Qi Gong. I asked her to explain TRE in relation to addiction.

Unexpressed emotions and feelings held within the body through fear, possibly through being subjected to danger, will impact our reactions and behaviour in our adult lives. We may think that we react normally, but because we are heavily traumatised, our decisions may not be the safest ones with regards to our health and wellbeing. This is Post Traumatic Stress Disorder (PTSD).

Qi Gong, pronounced Chee Kung, originates from China and is an ancient self-healing movement meditation. Spontaneous internal movements, which are the essence of Qi Gong, can often induce involuntary shaking or tremors when the body holds too much tension. Once triggered, the body will start shaking and releasing deeply held trauma and tension, thus restoring the body back to its natural harmonious state.

This is a reaction which is directly connected to our Central Nervous System and our 'Fight, Flight or Freeze' reflex, which we have learned to suppress, in order to survive and cope with overwhelm. It is an involuntary tremor, vibration or trembling which is triggered by the Core or Psoas muscles. This practice eases the stress on the hormone-releasing glands, allowing them to restore and to self-regulate, which in turn restores the entire body to a more balanced state. Mammals do this naturally.

It is not enough to provide talk therapies; the body needs to be able to release these held tensions too. When I realised just how powerful spontaneous Qi Gong was, I sought out courses offered by TRE Global, headed by Dr David Berceli, and became a qualified Provider in 2015.

Nadia Smith www.truetoourroots.co.uk

Chapter 16
THE SOBER HEART

Relationships

One of the biggest areas of resistance to staying alcohol-free is the reaction of others. When your partner is your drinking buddy, it's possible that you have been drinking together throughout your whole relationship. Alcohol is like the glue that sticks you together, and when it's taken away, you can feel as though the whole essence of your connection is threatened.

I played it down in the early weeks. My husband obviously noticed I was choosing to drink alcohol-free drinks, but we didn't discuss it. I can't say I did that consciously, but not having to explain myself or debate with anyone else helped me get through the difficult period.

It was interesting though to watch my husband watch me! Over time if he wanted a G&T and we didn't have any G, he would say, 'I'll try one of your alcohol-free alternatives'. I started making him 'pimped' drinks, and he absolutely loved the Sea Arch Botanical with a sprig of rosemary or a frozen berry dropped in it. After about 9 months of me not drinking, he suddenly said, 'I don't think I will bother with alcohol. What's the point when this alcohol-free stuff is so good?'

There was none of the pomp and ceremony, fragility or angst that came with my ditching the booze. For him it was a quick simple decision. I've since discovered it's very common for your partner to see the change in you, and want to experience it for themselves. Obviously, trying to cajole them, shame them or force them to stop won't work. (If the boot had been on the other foot and my husband had been nagging me to stop, I would have been incensed and probably have drunk even more.) So lead by example, but *do* remember this is your thing. It's non-negotiable and you are doing it for you.

One of my clients knew she needed to stop drinking. She had anxiety, felt bloated, overweight and angry with herself, but she really valued her weekends when she and her husband would sit on their deck at their lakeside home (sounds idyllic, doesn't it), drinking champagne together as the sun set.

Somehow, we have all glamorised alcohol so that we actually believe it's what's in the glass that is important rather than the company, the surroundings, the friendship, the occasion. Over time she was able to see that being in her 'happy place', having conversations with her husband and feeling relaxed were the important factors, and yes she wanted a nice, grown-up drink in her glass – a mug of tea or an orange juice certainly wouldn't be the same experience – but when she found a fabulous alcohol-free fizz and a kombucha that looked exactly the same, in the same lovely flute glass, she was able to realise that she wasn't missing anything, she was only gaining.

That's not to say that problems won't arise. I've heard from people who are furious when their partner carries on drinking. They notice whole sentences being repeated, they get tired and want to stop the party much earlier, then get worried they will be labelled 'boring'. Falling into bed with someone who reeks of booze can feel very off-putting. Then there's the question of how your drinking partner feels; one woman said her husband, a real wine buff, asked her in an incredulous voice when she was going to 'stop this silliness and start drinking again'. He implied that she was no fun sober. Actually, it's the drinkers who become boring really quite quickly!

I didn't share what I was going through because I was feeling shame and guilt. If I had my time again, I would have got support much earlier. I do recommend that you let your partner know what you are doing. Ask for the support you need. It may be important to remove alcohol from the home; make it clear that you don't want to be offered alcohol or pressurised into going into social occasions for a while. Explain that this is your thing, it's important to you, but you don't want to discuss it or debate – just yet.

Sober sex

Many of us when we quit the booze, find the idea of sex nerve-racking, even traumatic. In many cases, we have *never* had sober sex! If you started drinking as a teenager and have always drunk, then the absolute clarity and presence that comes with sobriety may never be something you have experienced, and you will become much more aware of the physical act, and your own naked body.

And, if you partner has been drinking, you have the way their alcohol breath smells to deal with. This can be tricky and sometimes a turn-off.

Check out Tawny Lara, who is a podcaster and writes on sexuality and sex and is known as a 'Sober Sexpert' – www.tawnylara.com.

If you are a young sober person navigating the dating scene, I strongly recommend you get connected with one of the great groups aimed at young people such as Millie Gooch's Sober Girl Society.

LGBT readers should check out Proud and Sober, which is run by Scott Pearson.

Men wanting advice on all aspects of sobriety, including sex and relationships, should check out Lee Davy and his team of coaches at 1000 Days Sober – www.1000dayssober.com

More mature readers might be interested in the work of Lucy Blenkinsopp, menopause expert and a coach for mid-life women. She has a theory on what can cause low sex drive in mid-life and that we should have a complete rethink about sex:

> Perhaps it is not just that we have gone off it, it is that we are bored to death of it. We need to inject some sort of excitement or change into it, because if you have been having sex with the same partner for years on end, then why wouldn't it get boring? I also believe, bedtime is the worst time for sex, most of us are

just too tired. I think afternoon sex is a much better idea and preferably not in the bedroom!

Mid-life women need to get brave and bold and start saying, 'Do you think we should try this or that? Let's go to a sex shop and buy some toys together.'

I hear many women say that their libido is low, but Lucy says that's because they haven't had an orgasm for ages. The less you have, the less you want – and the more you have, the more you want. So why not try and fix it?

Some older women find sex painful because of the lack of oestrogen and some may need testosterone. If so, a women's health expert is a good place to start.

I also asked Lucy about where body image and self-esteem fits in – and not surprisingly she said women become very disconnected with their bodies during and after menopause, especially if their bodies have changed shape and the quality of skin is changing. Sober and naked? That does sounds scary.

The good news is that this can be overcome and there is plenty of information and advice available.

Parenting

There is a saying you will be familiar with: No regrets. Sadly, I do have some. I regret not ditching the booze sooner so that I could be fully present for my children when they were young. It makes me feel emotional just writing that sentence, and when Clare Pooley described in *The Sober Diaries* how she would race through bedtime stories, missing out lines, hoping her children wouldn't notice, to get to the cold glass of wine that was waiting, it really resonated with me. I wasn't ever rolling drunk in front of them, apart from one occasion when, according to my teenage son I was 'over the top' at a family party and embarrassed him and his friends. The reality is, though, that children don't like their parents to be intoxicated, it can lead to unpredictability and insecurity.

The whole wine o'clock, drinking culture is a problem in the UK. Alcohol is seen as the social glue that bonds parents, it's there at the baby shower, at the PTA meeting and, if you drop your child off at someone's house for a play date, you will probably weigh up whether you might be friends by the wine you are offered. We've all been there, dropping off the kids and greeted by: 'Lovely to meet you. Want a cuppa, or something stronger?' 'Of course,' you reply. 'It would be rude not to!' I've lost count of the times I ended up chatting away about nothing much, drinking copious amounts of wine while the kids played, then having to call a taxi to take us home because I was over the limit. Shameful.

I guess I was seduced by media messaging around alcohol. Wine was the only treat, the way to feel grown-up and worthwhile again after a gruelling day of childcare and what feels like isolation. Of course, I also read with glee the many articles telling me that wine was good for me. Obviously, I ignored the small print that covered their backsides ('in moderation'). I just read the bit that said resveratrol (found in the skin of grapes) is good for the heart. As Catherine Gray writes so eloquently in *The Unexpected Joy of Being Sober*: 'Drinking red wine because it's good for you is like choosing a burger for the gherkin.'

For those of us with children and grandchildren, know that your sobriety is the best gift you can ever give to them. They will notice that you are calmer, more reasoned and kinder. Having said that, I've spoken to many sober parents who say their kids get away with less. Children see your weak spot and ask for stuff when you are too merry to care. I know that I am a much better parent to my teenagers now and it's genuinely one of the best, most responsible reasons to ditch the booze.

When I was only a couple of weeks sober, my son, then 19, had to work late at a café. Just before midnight, he rang me and said, 'I don't suppose Dad can pick me up?' It was only ever my husband who could do those late-night trips, I had always been drinking, and in fact would usually be sloshed by 10 p.m. I was proud to be able to say: 'I'll come and get you now.'

I was wiping away the tears of joy as I got in the car – tears of sadness that I hadn't been there for the kids before and tears of joy for the fact that I was free and would be happy to be stopped by the police for a routine check.

As time has gone on, of course, the novelty of being called out at all hours has worn off a little, but the feeling of absolute joy, knowing you are present and available for your kids, is incredible.

I asked some of the Sober Club members to share their thoughts on how being sober makes them a better parent. Here are a few comments:

- *I have far more patience and don't get stressed like I used to. Also when I take away their gadgets at night I can remember where I put them in the morning.*
- *My child is a big driver for me staying sober She is three now and so full of questions and life. By not drinking I sleep better, and this gives me the energy that a three-year-old needs their parent to have. I don't want her to grow up in a 'snappy' household, but a happy household.*
- *My grown-up daughters look at me with pride and my grandchildren give me 1000 reasons to stay sober.*
- *Wow, what an apt question for me this morning! My son came into the bedroom last night at 10 whilst I was reading and started confiding to me about his worries regarding his university exam results. We lay there till late, discussing it all. Never could I have listened and helped at that time before. It felt fab that I was really 'there for him.'*
- *I have so much more patience overall. My kids are young, so get up very early – that was sooo hard with hangovers, which meant I was very short tempered in the mornings, and made me feel incredibly guilty. Now we have lovely peaceful mornings.*
- *Huge change! I look back with regret. My daughter saw me with a wine glass while I was cooking dinner, after dinner, and carrying one to bed most nights. I was never really 'available' for her to talk to. What teenager wants to talk to a drunk parent? I couldn't remember anything we talked about anyway. Fast forward to now...I have shown her that you can make changes in your life.*

For those of us with young teenagers, how do we teach them about alcohol? Just because we have ditched the drink doesn't mean we can steam in and prohibit them from ever trying alcohol. That's likely to lead to more rebellion. It's really important to keep a channel of communication. Dr Aric Sigman is a psychologist, educational lecturer and author of *Alcohol Nation: how to protect our children from today's drinking culture* and *Body Wars: why body dissatisfaction is at epidemic proportions and how we can fight back*. He believes that children really do take notice of what we do and what we say. Despite them seeming to eschew every view and belief their parents have, studies show that in fact parental influence is massive. He says we should absolutely share our own stories with our children and teach them the truth around alcohol. If nothing else Aric says we can point them to the research that tells us that our brains aren't fully developed until we are around 21. Aric offers educational talks in schools, and when he spoke at my kids' school when they were around 14 and 15, he spoke very much in their language, reminding the boys that if they drink too much alcohol an erection won't be possible. Beer isn't called Brewers Droop for no reason!

Wendy Laban is a Sober Club member who is now two years sober. She has – wait for it – seven children, and she has this to say:

> For me, the most powerful change is being able to model a healthy relationship with alcohol within the family home. Sure, I talk about my thoughts and feelings around this addictive drug that is still so normalised in our society, but mainly it's the power of my unspoken behaviour – I've had a tough day and I don't reach for a glass of wine, it's my birthday and I don't need Prosecco to make it fun, I sleep well and wake up able to honour my commitments to others. There's the patience, time and understanding that being sober also brings to parenting, and these are wonderful things to now have, but for me the greatest pride comes from living an alcohol-free life in front of their very eyes instead of reinforcing, daily, the widely held myth that we need this stuff to be happy, successful and 'grown-up'.

Friendship

The opposite of addiction is connection.

It has been said so many times! The phrase was made famous by Johann Hari in his TEDx Talk 'Everything you think you know about addiction is wrong'.

We all need friends, and yet in our society far more emphasis is put on romantic relationships. There is a lot of research on childhood and adolescent friendships but not so much on how close friendships are beneficial for us as we age. They don't just stay strong by accident, though. We need to nurture friendships and show our appreciation for those important people in our lives who are there for us no matter what.

The whole issue of friends has become so blurred with social media that we may have literally thousands of 'friends' on Facebook – but would any of them actually lend you a fiver? The truth of it is, most of us have a handful of real friends – what I call 2 a.m. friends. Someone who will come out at 2 a.m. for you if you are in trouble. Some of us find it hard to think of friends who would do that; their immediate thought is, 'I couldn't ask anyone.'

Most of us don't want to feel as though we are a burden to others, so we don't allow ourselves to be held by friends even when we need comfort. So turn the question around and ask: Is there anyone for whom you are a 2 a.m. friend? I would go and rescue a friend without question if they needed it; there are a few people I would do that for. And you?

The whole concept of the BFF (Best Friend Forever) can be tricky. The friend you were close to throughout childhood and perhaps early teens might turn into an absolute bitch/arse when she/he meets their life partner, who happens to disapprove of you. One of my closest friends who I'd known for over 15 years literally disappeared out of my life when she got engaged to a guy who just didn't like me, that's the long and short of it. It hurt me – in truth, it still does – and it felt like betrayal, but she made her choice.

If your friendships were formed around drinking, it can be hard when one person stops if the other doesn't. I am ashamed to say I used to avoid getting too close to non-drinkers. I gravitated towards those who loved a drink, probably to validate my own drinking, and when I finally stopped, there was some navigating to do, because suddenly it became a 'thing'. I couldn't just meet a friend for drinks as I had before, because there would be all the questions around my decision to quit.

Good, conscious friendships are worth holding on to: I still have friends I have known for years, though I rarely see them. We live at opposite ends of the UK and are busy, but when we catch up or spend time together we really can pick up where we left off. The bonds are strong and my friends have, in an odd way, helped me to define my sense of self. They have shaped me, in different ways. One friend still loves her alcohol, but genuinely doesn't believe she has a problem. She has an off switch. She totally respects my decision not to drink and is happy to come over for mocktails or alcohol-free drinks. It's not awkward because there is a mutual respect.

Don't let your decision to be alcohol-free get in the way. You wouldn't judge or dismiss a friend for making their own dietary choices, hobbies or travel, even if they are different to yours. Focus on what's going on for you and don't try and make it right for the other person. Over time, friends may start to be curious for themselves about giving up the booze, especially if they see a positive difference in you.

Of course, you may find that some friendships don't make it. People can literally feel betrayed that you have chosen not to drink, but that's their thing.

Most of us have chosen our friends because they have similar interests, or you like their qualities, but of course people change, and over time if your friends no longer share your values or interests it can get tricky. What we all need is friends who support us, cheer us up when we are down, give us a hug and spur us on to reach our goals even when we feel nervous and inadequate.

So, how do we find sober friends? When I ditched the booze, I knew no one at all who had been through the same experience, it felt daunting. I joined the Club Soda Facebook group and eventually plucked up the courage to go to a lunch meet-up locally. I was so nervous, I literally walked around the car park for fifteen minutes before walking in! Of course, I had nothing to be nervous about;

former drinkers who have 'seen the light' tend to be great fun. I have since made so many sober friends and feel totally enriched. Being sober bonds us together.

Online friendships can be of value too, of course. Many of the Sober Club members will never meet, but still feel very close to one another through online connection and activities.

For some people, especially young people, FOMO is massive. It's the fear of missing out on social occasions, fear of losing their friends or not being accepted in social circles. All is not lost: within groups of teens and millennials there is a whole growing trend of sobriety. I asked Millie Gooch, who runs Sober Girl Society, for her view:

If you tell someone that you've stopped drinking at any age, they will expect you to have a shocking tale of rock-bottom horror, but when you tell someone that you've stopped drinking in your twenties, they're almost disappointed when you don't. The truth is, most people find it hard to understand why anyone would want to stop drinking in their partying prime, and the expectation is that something must have gone terribly wrong to prompt such a decision.

I quit alcohol when I was 26, which means coming in at under a decade, my drinking career was relatively short-lived. Still, I managed to pack a lot in, which meant that by the time I stopped, I had still suffered my fair share of mystery bruises, hangovers from hell and nights lost to boozy blackouts. By February 2018, my self-esteem was on the floor and weekend hangovers started to take a more permanent toll on my mental health. My nights were becoming harder to piece together and I soon realised that drinking was now my entire identity. I was the drunk girl, the one who usually flashed her knickers and had to spend the next day making grovelling apologies to her friends. One day, on a particularly queasy hangover, I downloaded *The Unexpected Joy of Being Sober* by Catherine Gray and never looked back. No rock bottom, just a realisation that alcohol was holding me back from living the life that I really wanted.

Being a young woman and navigating everything, from dating to her mate's weddings, without a drop can be hard – which is why, seven months in to my sobriety, I started Sober Girl Society, one of the first Instagram platforms for millennial women navigating an alcohol-free life. Since then I have done so much, from launching a boozeless brunch series to working with universities to change drinking culture amongst students.

Despite the fact I'm now nearly 30, I'm often asked why I believe the younger generation are drinking less, and whilst I think there are many reasons, I think a widening conversation around mental health is one of the most important. I also think social media allows those of us living fun, fulfilled lives without alcohol to show others it is possible. Sobriety is not a trend, but platforms like Instagram make it easier than ever to find others who happily living life sober and will follow their lead.

Millie Gooch, *The Sober Girl Society Handbook*

Self-love

One of my favourite books is *I Heart Me: The Science of Self Love* by prolific author David Hamilton, who has made his name talking about kindness. In this book David, a former biochemist, fuses science with self-help to offer powerful strategies for loving yourself. It isn't about boosting your ego, though. Far from it. The messages are for those who have, in truth, probably loathed themselves for years; they may not have gone as far as self-harming, but the negative talk is constant, even if not voiced out loud.

We all have the Inner Critic, the voice telling us that we aren't enough, that we don't look right, that we are too fat, too thin, too old, unworthy.

Most of us, despite being enlightened and aware of the concept of self-loving, actually find it quite hard to apply it to ourselves. I remember the words of Cheryl Richardson, leading author and life coach: if we spoke out loud what we were thinking when we look in the mirror, and a child were in the room, we'd be accused of abuse!

There is a lot of talk right now about kindness, about the benefits of offering random acts of kindness to others, but not so much about being 'self-kind' – at least not when it goes deep. We talk about self-care, and the need for taking some time out, walking in nature, having a nice bath, lighting a candle, indulging in some chocolate but we don't often really look into what being 'self-kind' means. The truth of it is, we are much harder on ourselves than we would be on others; we see qualities in others, we forgive them, we cheer them on even when they have messed up, but we rarely afford the same acceptance of ourselves.

I was speaking at the same event as David Hamilton when he was launching *I Heart Me*, and was surprised to hear him say that he didn't actually love himself. Not really, not deep down, and it was something he needed to address.

That really resonated with me, but it felt too awkward to admit it then. Everything on the surface was fine. I was a successful author, with four beautiful kids and a career I loved, and I knew I was able to inspire others with my work around holistic living. But if you'd hooked me up to a lie detector and asked: 'Do you appreciate and value yourself?', the answer would be have been a resounding 'Hell, no!'

If you had questioned me at length, I suppose I would have said I thought self-loving was something others felt, but not me. The whole 'not enough' mantra ran through me like a line through a stick of rock.

What changed? I quit drinking alcohol. Unrelated, right? No, turns out it was the missing piece of my holistic living jigsaw.

Hindsight is a wonderful thing. Looking back, I can see that alcohol was keeping me small, taking away my spirit (literally), keeping me at a lower vibration, and stopping me from being able to love myself.

At around eight months clear of booze, I wrote about the benefits I had found. In addition to the usual – clearer skin, better sleep, etc. – I wrote that the biggest and most surprising benefit of all is that I felt more stable and less chaotic, and I began to be self-kind. So – yes, I can finally say it – I love myself.

I Heart Me. There is definitely no puffed-up ego, no sense of being holier than thou, and I'm definitely not better than you. I am probably more grateful than I have ever been.

David's books have been published by publishing company Hay House, and founder Louise Hay, dubbed The Queen of New Age by the *New York Times*, is a strong advocate of self-loving. Louise believes in affirmations and is a great advocate of what she calls Mirror Work – looking in the mirror several times a day and saying 'I love you, [add your name]'. Just try it a few times, and you will realise how tricky it can feel. I remember being in the audience when she spoke and invited us all to go the bathroom in the break and say: 'I love you' at your own reflection in the mirror. Wow, that was uncomfortable! Louise used to carry around a tiny mirror in her bra so that she could whip it out at any point and remind herself.

Despite being an author who was promoting self-loving and self-care, I couldn't believe in any of it for myself. Over time I became 'self-loving and self-care curious' – and that's what I'd urge you to do too.

Look in the mirror and say, 'I love you.'

I encourage you to look in the mirror often – but not in the name of vanity, or to worry about your wrinkles, commiserate about greying hairs, or pull faces to tighten your jaw, just look in the mirror in order to be appreciative, to show love to yourself.

> Today I asked my body what she needed,
> Which is a big deal
> Considering my journey of
> Not Really Asking That Much.
>
> I thought she might need more water.
> Or protein.
> Or greens.
> Or yoga.
> Or supplements.
> Or movement.
>
> But as I stood in the shower
> Reflecting on her stretch marks,
> Her roundness where I would like flatness,
> Her softness where I would like firmness,

All those conditioned wishes
That form a bundle of
Never-Quite-Right-Ness,

She whispered very gently:
Could you just love me like this?

Hollie Holden www.hollieholden.me

Chapter 17
THE SOBER BODY

Look and feel younger

I remember feeling very anxious indeed about getting older. There aren't many women who relish their skin and hair becoming more dry, wrinkles appearing and everything going south, and I was fearful that I would just become a much worse version of who I was, especially the bits I didn't like. I could only imagine being bloated and looking grey in my late fifties and sixties, with zero energy. I was imagining hot flushes and memory losses, and these thoughts made me scared.

The truth is, ditching the booze makes you younger. It is literally the best antidote to ageing ever. Better than any HRT, youth elixir or Botox!

If you want to look and feel younger, I have the secret. Stop drinking alcohol. It's that simple. (You're welcome!)

> When it comes to getting older, my big brother believes that by the time you reach 50 you had the face you deserve!
>
> When I turned 50 it would be fair to say that I was beginning to look every one of my 50 years, including having suffered with rosacea for a number of years.

This was a combination of a stressful job working long hours, living a booze-filled expat life... in the sunshine in the Caribbean. Not to mention a long-standing habit of self-soothing and numbing with wine, often choosing wine over food at the end of a stressful day.

Exactly a month before my 51st birthday I gave up the booze – and what happened then was nothing short of a miracle in terms of anti-ageing.

No more puffiness or dark circles from lack of sleep and the tell-tale red complexion. Now replaced with clear skin and bright eyes and no longer needing to wear thick cover up makeup and my fair skin even tanned all over for the first time. Yes, tanned brown legs – who would have thought it!

My only regret is that I did not give up the dreaded poison years earlier!

Dominique

You may see a photo of me and wonder if I am a little delusional thinking that I am looking younger, but who cares? I feel better, I no longer hate myself and I have masses of vitality.

I remember hearing Dr Christiane Northrup talking about ageing when she was promoting her excellent book *Goddesses Never Age*. She said: 'Be careful how you speak to yourself. Don't say: "I'm having a senior moment" just because you forgot what you walked into a room to get. Just see your own brain as an overloaded computer, perhaps you just need a reboot.'

It's not just me who believes giving up the booze makes us younger. Sober Club member Wendy Laban writes:

I didn't realise how old alcohol was making me feel until I completely removed it from my life in my late forties. What I thought were the inescapable characteristics of ageing, were largely just the mental and physical representations of a mind and body fully held back from its healthy potential by alcohol.

I gave booze far too much power, space and influence in my life. I used it to try and treat myself, to soothe, to celebrate, to numb any uncomfortable emotions and to try and relax. All it did was wreck my sleep patterns, my self-worth, my passion for personal growth, my bank balance and my zest for life.

No more!

Now two and a half years alcohol-free, I'm feeling energised and excited to try new things. I've started running and I feel fit and toned. My varicose veins have calmed right down, and I no longer have a redness to my cheeks. My nails grow long without breaking and my teeth are whiter. My hair seems thicker and definitely more shiny. My skin glows and my eyes are bright. I can concentrate much better and my thinking is clear and sharp. Best of all, my sense of self-worth just keeps on growing.

All these things make me feel youthful and joyful. I'm motivated every single day to carry on discovering my best ever sober life.

PAWS

I hate being a party pooper, but I feel I must share with you the news about PAWS.

After the initial euphoria, and the buzz of ditching the booze and starting to love your life, some of us can 'hit the wall' and end up feeling blue. Up to two years into sobriety (ouch!), we can suffer from PAWS. I'd never heard of it either, and there is nothing cute or puppy-like about it: it stands for Post-Acute Withdrawal Symptoms. And it feels as though something has come back to bite you on the bum, just when you least expect it. I had assumed that after the initial ten days or so, when our body detoxes the physical effects of the alcohol, it would be plain sailing. Sadly, some of us experience a second stage.

It's important to know that it's temporary, and especially if you are prepared, it can be managed. It will pass! Former drinkers often have lots of other issues on their plate. They may not crave alcohol, but suddenly and seemingly out of the blue they can feel as though they are on a roller coaster. Stress can trigger it and so can flashbacks of something that happened during their 'drinking career', which triggers feelings of anxiety, of guilt and shame.

You may start to experience cravings to drink again, even though you thought you'd knocked that on the head! You may have anxiety, low energy levels, irritability, mood swings, all those rubbish feelings you thought you'd seen the back of.

So, what can we do to support ourselves through all of this? As I've said before, a lot comes down to that crucial balance of brain chemistry; we need to start naturally producing endorphins, and we need that balance of serotonin, GABA and dopamine. So a quick recap:

Eating well really helps – you need good nutrients and superfoods.
Practice good self-care – you need good restorative sleep and exercise.
Connect with like-minded people who can support and encourage you.
Set boundaries – if certain people drain your energy, stay away from them.
Write down your thoughts and feelings in a journal. It helps.
'Switch off' for a while; try listening to a meditation or hypnosis audio.
Write gratitude lists – celebrate the good things.
Be self-kind – loving yourself just as you are is so important. (At least try!)

And most importantly, never suffer in silence, seek help if you need it.

PAWS will pass, I promise you.

Mood-altering drinks

Can drinks be spiritual?

There has been much talked about the mood-altering effects of alcohol, for those who want to step away from their mundane lives and enter a different space if just for a while. The whole concept is flawed, of course. What we really want surely is a life so wonderful that we don't need to step away.

We know that many millennials are choosing to avoid booze and that has to be a good thing. Sober raves and clubs are happening, where sugar, flavourings, chemicals and, of course, alcohol are off the menu. We find superfoods, cacao, plant-based foods and alcohol-free artisan drinks alongside the banging dancefloor. Should we think of any drinks as mood enhancers?

One brand regularly rocking up to conscious events is Senser Spirits, who claim that harnessing the transformative power of nature 'brings us to our senses'. By opening up a whole new realm of discovery, we can inspire a deeper connection between people, plants and the planet.

The founders of the brand are James and Vanessa Jacoby, plant alchemists who say:

> Our specially crafted blends of active natural botanicals, are designed so that a 50 ml serve delivers a significant adaptogenic dosage. You can have them neat, over ice or with a mixer. They're crafted to move your mind and mood and encourage drinkers to turn away from alcohol and towards nature to get their needs met.

There is a range of three, consisting of Power, Love and Joy, because that's typically why we drink alcohol – apparently!

In a nutshell:

POWER
EFFECTS: Sage brings calm grounded presence, gotu kola and Siberian ginseng cause a rousing empowerment of the body's systems as you get centred and on your game.
TASTING NOTES: A sophisticated blend crafted with orange, spiced cacao and vanilla, finishing with a complex herbal smoked orange bitter.

LOVE
EFFECTS: Tulsi, ashwaghanda, hibiscus and passionflower produce a state of relaxed serenity, facilitating harmony and

ease as you wind down, cosy with a loved one, or enjoy with friends.

TASTING NOTES: Sensual florals, rose and bergamot woven with spiced aronia, luscious lime flower, cardamom and hawthorn, with a long bittersweet spiced berry finish.

JOY

EFFECTS: This joy bringer blend includes schisandra and gingko to clear the mind and energise the body, while damiana and nutmeg raise the spirit as you celebrate life and party into the night.

TASTING NOTES: Fresh citrus tones, elderflower and lavender heights, then sweet quince, exuberant schizandra berry and a stimulating balanced length of salty sour acidity.

And here's how to really experience them –

Listen
As your pour, close your eyes and listen for the double shot.

Look
Look closely at the liquid and sense for the plants that are still vibrant and alive.

Smell
Breathe deep, filling the entire body with scents.

Taste
Sip slowly and immerse the tastebuds, savouring the height, breadth and length.

Feel
Tune in. Be transported. And why not!

James and Vanessa Jacoby www.senserspirits.com

The power of plants

It's only when you become aware of the importance of nutrition that you start to realise the power of plants. Of course, we know that we should eat more fruit and veg, but what about herbs, spices and adaptogens?

If you're new to all of this and the closest you've come to it is enjoying a cup of herbal tea, never fear, there is a whole world to discover! One of my favourite brands is Pukka Herbs.

Its in-house research team works with leading universities and medical schools to advance understanding of the role organic herbs can take in nurturing healthier, happier lives. From investigations around turmeric and bowel cancer to trials exploring ashwagandha and mental health, they fund world-leading research to bring the wonder of herbs into our modern world.

Euan MacLennan, Herbal and Sustainability Director, says:

> For centuries plants have supported our health and wellbeing. ... In more concentrated forms, they also form the foundations of medicines we use to prevent or treat illness. We harness the active compounds within plants and employ them in general practices and hospitals around the world. Interestingly, the more we understand about plants and medicine, the more we realise that they not only alleviate or prevent disease, but they also actively contribute to our wellbeing and quality of life.

Ashwagandha is a herb that has been used in traditional Indian healing (Ayurveda) for centuries and was considered to bring mental strength and calm nervous energy. Clinical research has shown that, through its action on chemical messengers in the brain, ashwagandha may harbour great promise as a treatment for stress and anxiety, two conditions that contribute hugely to health outcomes and life choices.

Cinnamon, a common culinary herb, has an amazing history of medicinal use. Having been used to treat dysentery, cholera and many other serious conditions, we still prescribe it for soothing upset stomachs and to ease digestion. Research shows that cinnamon may lower blood glucose levels and improve the role of insulin in managing sugar within the blood. Another herb, *Gymnema sylvestre*, called the 'sugar destroyer' in traditional medicine, even blocks sweet receptors in the mouth, meaning that you cannot taste the sweetness of chocolate!

Turmeric is one herb that stands out in terms of its potential to support long-term cardiovascular, digestive and mental health. It can be taken as a supplement or in home cooking to help you combat some of the major causes of chronic and age-related diseases.

Euan MacLennan www.pukkaherbs.com/

While we are on the topic of plants, it's always good to hear from a doctor who is totally invested in the holistic picture. Dr Gemma Newman is known as The Plant Power Doctor, and recommends real food as the antidote to ill health! Sounds obvious but it's a rare thing! Gemma says:

Too much alcohol can cause a myriad of health issues, if it had been invented more recently it would most likely be illegal. Why? It boils down to the first and most toxic metabolite of alcohol – acetaldehyde. Acetaldehyde reacts with DNA to form cancer-promoting compounds. In addition, highly reactive, oxygen-containing molecules that are generated during pathways of alcohol metabolism can damage your DNA, making you more prone to things like breast cancer too.

What can we do when we want to minimise the harm? Nature can come to the rescue! Fortunately, the polyphenols and antioxidants in fruits and veggies are not just confined to red grapes. These little miracle workers are present in many fruits, vegetables, herbs and spices and can potentially minimise hangovers but also, more crucially, reduce long-term harms of over consumption of alcohol. They help your body break down acetaldehyde by ramping up your body's production of antioxidants and enzymes that can break it down. Sulforaphane (from veggies like broccoli, cauliflower and kale) quercetin (from onions, green tea and berries) and curcumin (good old turmeric) may improve alcohol metabolism, alleviate hangover symptoms and help your liver to do the important task of detoxification.

Give your body the best chance of building your body parts that function normally and improve your long-term health. The best foods to minimise long term risk of cancer (on top of ditching or minimising the booze) are fruits, veggies whole grains and legumes like green beans, chickpeas and lentils. A hangover bean burrito never looked so appealing!

Dr Gemma Newman www.plantpowerdoctor.com

Loving your liver after booze

I had a dull ache around my liver area for years when I was drinking. Once I had it checked with an ultrasound scan which showed nothing, but a little nagging voice told me there was something wrong. Lo and behold, a short time after I stopped drinking, and with a little TLC, the pain went. Of course, I will never know if that's what was going on, but I suspect my liver was grateful I gave it a chance to heal!

The truth is the liver can repair, and there are ways we can nurture it after years of drinking.

Recognising the key role that liver plays in digestion, I decided to introduce more different foods into my diet.

Foods that help to nourish the liver

Eat sour foods such as artichoke to nourish the liver. Lemons have a diuretic effect, you can drink the juice of a whole lemon in hot water first thing in the morning and add a whole lemon (unpeeled) to your juice, but make sure it's organic and unwaxed. Yep, they are more expensive, but think how much money you are saving by not drinking booze!

Vegetables that support the liver are the leafy green ones, so eat as much broccoli, kale, spinach, watercress and rocket as you like. Vitamin C is also important to help calm inflammation, so once again that's leafy green vegetables, peppers, and citrus fruit. Omega-3 is also essential, found in oily fish, eggs, nuts, seeds and olive oil. B vitamins are also important, found again in nuts, seeds, eggs, and in meat, cheese and beans.

Because repairing and looking after your liver is so important after ditching the booze, I asked naturopath Katie Ruane for advice: 'The first thing to do is to give your liver at least 12 hours overnight with no food or drinks to metabolise. This gives the liver time to repair, remove toxins from the body and also helps the body re-regulate blood sugar levels so the sugar cravings reduce.'

Katie also shared these two recipes:

Watercress and Rocket Salad

Watercress and rocket (also known as arugula) are 'bitter greens', which means that they help get the digestive system ready to digest food by stimulating the pancreas to produce enzymes which break down the food. They also help the liver produce bile that is stored and released from the gall bladder.

> 1 × bag rocket
> 1 × bag watercress
> pumpkin seeds, toasted
> ½ lemon
> extra virgin olive oil
> English mustard (optional)
> raspberry vinegar (optional)
> salt (optional)
> sugar (optional)

Get a bag of watercress and a bag of rocket, then wash, dry and put in a bowl. For the dressing, drizzle with extra virgin olive oil and the juice of ½ lemon.

For an alternative dressing, mix together 30 ml of extra virgin olive oil, ½ teaspoon of English mustard, 1 tablespoon of raspberry vinegar, a pinch of salt and ½ teaspoon of sugar. Mix together vigorously with a spoon or a little whisk. Try it and then add in more of the above to get it to the flavour that you like.

Sprinkle plain or dry toasted pumpkin seeds on the top for a bit of crunch. To dry toast the seeds, set a pan over medium heat for about a couple of minutes, or until warm, then add the seeds and shake them around or stir. It can take around 5 minutes for them to toast. If you can see that they are burning/smell burnt, remove from the pan immediately.

Add to the salad bowl.

Chia Seed Pudding

This pudding needs to be refrigerated, so make a couple of hours before you want to eat it. This is high in protein, fat, fibre and a bit of sugar to help with the cravings.

> 4–5 (tablespoons) chia seeds
> 400 ml coconut milk, unsweetened
> 4 (squares) 85% dark chocolate (optional)
> plain, unsalted mixed nuts, or a favourite nut of your choice
> raspberries

If you like rich and creamy puddings, use coconut milk from a tin. If you prefer lighter puddings, use coconut milk from a carton.

Get an eating bowl (not a mixing bowl) and mix together 4 tablespoons chia seeds and coconut milk and leave to soak for 10–15 minutes. Give it a stir and if it's too watery, add in another 1 tablespoon of seeds, and if it's too thick, add in more coconut milk or water.

Once it's set to the consistency you like, grate in some of the chocolate – if you have a really sweet/chocolate tooth, melt 4 squares of the dark chocolate and add that to the coconut milk before mixing in the chia seeds.

Sprinkle over some of the nuts and some raspberries.

Pop in the fridge for a couple of hours before eating.

Katie Ruane www.thefamilynaturopath.co.uk

Additional ways to support your liver

Here are a couple of more tips I can share with you to help your liver.

- Katie Brindle, a practitioner of Chinese medicine and the founder of the Hayo'u Method (see www.hayoumethod.com), offered an analogy of going on holiday and coming back to a pile of mail (perhaps not entirely appropriate these days, what with email, but you get the drift). If we decided we were too exhausted and left the pile to deal with later, it wouldn't go away. And when we go on holiday again, the same thing happens. It's a bit like that when we stop drinking; the liver suddenly finds that the abuse has stopped and now is a good time to go back and finally deal with the issues that have built up.

There are some simple liver boosters. Acupuncture and acupressure can be good for a liver imbalance (see resources) and you can try some simple self-massage on the right points. Gua Sha massage is often used in Chinese medicine, a therapeutic healing technique that involves a round edged tool, traditionally made form metal or jade. Brindle suggests using the massage tool along the liver points (starting at the big toe and moving up the body along the inside of the leg) to help stimulate this area. Press and stroke the skin until redness appears, a sign of increased circulation, which can clear inflammation by increasing blood flow to the surface of the skin.

- Breathe! It sounds very obvious, but we do need to take time to breathe – properly.

    Make sure you fully breathe out, especially first thing in the morning and then take five deep inhalations. As you slowly breathe out each time, bring your energy downwards and imagine that you are 'smiling with your liver'. You've seen the film *Eat Pray Love*? The medicine man swore by it!

- Make sure you drink plenty of water.

Fitness

I've heard of people who ditch the booze and become fitness fanatics. It's not a bad cross addiction to develop, but as with anything it's best to have a balanced relationship with exercise.

This bit isn't the easiest for me to write because I absolutely can't lead by example. I did nothing more than walking and a bit of yoga in the first few months of ditching the booze and probably felt a bit sorry for myself as I piled a few pounds of weight on, rather than losing them. However, when the 'pink cloud of euphoria' appeared and I settled into my happy place as a sober person, I did get back into the aspects of fitness I had originally enjoyed. There is no doubt whatsoever that moving your body is critically important and exercising can release some of those happy feel good hormones that we are lacking in the early days of not drinking. Going for a walk can literally lift your mood and a 30-minute brisk walk while swinging your arms (while listening to a podcast) will be very beneficial.

Whatever type of exercise you choose, it has to be the one you love, it's all about mindset.

I am not a fan of gyms or even gym workouts, but if you are – go for it! During lockdown in April 2020, my teenage son who is a personal trainer used our living room as his gym to offer training sessions on Zoom. Quite frankly I was exhausted just listening to him encouraging his clients to 'push through it, squeeze their butt, go for the burn'.

I much prefer dance and have loved getting along to sober raves such as Morning Gloryville, where you can enjoy movement for its own sake and no one cares. I love Nia dance, a blend of nine different movement forms, and then there's 5Rhythms and Biodanza.

I am a huge *Strictly* fan (who isn't?) and would love to try some ballroom dancing sessions, but sadly don't have a partner who will join me. The next best thing is Fitsteps, which was devised by one of the choreographers for *Strictly*. It's all done without a partner, so you find yourself in a dance studio or a gym with a bunch of other people, shaking your booty, doing the American Smooth or the foxtrot to Meatloaf's 'I'd do anything for love' or Will.I.Am's 'I Like to Move It'. All styles are covered and you can dance in trainers – no sparkly Jimmy Choos needed!

There is, of course, a connection between moving our body and being our ideal weight, but it really isn't as simple as 'eat a doughnut, run a few miles – no weight gained'. Keilly Natalie Foster, founder of Fit Alcohol Free Coaching, says: 'I assumed I'd lose weight when I quit drinking, but nope, I gained 30 lb! Even though I'm a personal trainer, I didn't notice that I'd replaced drinking alcohol with eating sugar... It's often called addiction transfer.'

Keilly agrees that the main focus early in sobriety must be ditching the booze, and not on losing weight. It can take 3–12 months for everything to 'regulate'. After 6 months, she felt ready to tackle her weight, but couldn't face doing a restrictive diet:

> I started counting calories and ensuring I ate enough protein for my weight. This stabilised my blood sugar levels and gave me the flexibility to eat what I wanted within reason.
>
> I now teach this same approach to my clients using the 80/20 method (80% wholefoods, 20% junk), which enables them to enjoy takeaways, a bar of chocolate, etc, without feeling like they've fallen off track.

Keilly Natalie Foster www.Fitafcoaching.com

Yoga and pilates

I have been doing yoga for years, though truth be told, I'm not sure I am any better at it than when I started. Fortunately, it doesn't matter because yoga isn't in any way competitive; the whole idea is to work with your own body and mind.

Yoga is a good choice of exercise when you ditch the booze. It's good for bringing calm to the nervous system and, of course, it's great for breathing, stamina and relaxation. In truth there were days in the early weeks of sobriety when I felt exhausted and had a roller coaster of emotions. I attended my yoga classes (it was amazing not to feel dizzy doing the upside-down poses) and really embraced the corpse pose. I carry on doing yoga because I know it's good for me. I noticed that when I wasn't doing as much yoga during lockdown in 2020 I had a really sluggish digestion. Getting back on the yoga mat really made a difference, even for just a few simple stretches.

Ciara Jean Roberts is a naturopathic nutritionist and yoga teacher who believes that yoga is hugely beneficial especially as we age. She says that one of the key requirements to good health as we age is bone density and one of the many physical benefits of yoga is that weight bearing through the natural use of our own body is great news for the bones. So if it's good for bringing us calm when we are off the booze and for keeping us young, why not have a go! Find details of her classes and workshops at www.whollyaligned.com

Here's a taster for you to help you feel calm:

Lie flat on the floor, rest the hands on your belly and simply observe your breath moving in and out of your body. Spend 5–10 minutes like this. You should begin to feel calmer and more relaxed. Remember, yoga is very much about a whole feeling rather than just physical exercise. It is about a connection between your mind and your body.

Pilates is also fantastic if you find the right teacher. For a while, I was attending classes that I didn't enjoy. Squeezing my butt cheeks 40 times just didn't do it for me and I found I was looking at the clock, hoping the class would end! It doesn't have to be that way!

Pilates is an exercise technique developed by the late Joseph Pilates. There are 8 Principles: relaxation, breathing, core stability, alignment, concentration, co-ordination, flowing movements and stamina.

Pilates can really help the back if you do the right exercises for you and with good technique and alignment. It helps you strengthen your back muscles, and improve your posture, which is often a really good way to reduce back pain. The breathing, stretching and relaxation helps too. It also improves your core stability, strengthening your deep abdominal muscles that help you support your back as well as helping you become more toned.

Beverley Densham has been a Pilates expert for many years and now teaches Mindfulness Pilates which aims to deepen your practice of Pilates, while bringing the added benefits of extra relaxation and meditation during the class. Positive affirmations are also used to help with mindset.

There is a holistic element as well. You're encouraged to use essential oils in class, such as lavender for extra relaxation or eucalyptus oil to be refreshing and energising and help your breathing. You are taught to listen to your body rather than 'go for the burn'. The session ends with a deep relaxation and meditation to calm the mind and body.

Here are two exercises Beverley suggests you can safely try at home:

The Number 10 meditation

Lie on your back with your knees bent, on a mat or blanket folded into four with a cushion behind your head. Close your eyes. Take 10 breaths in and out – breathe in through your nose and as you exhale through your mouth relax. Relax more and more on each out breath.

Stretch your back

Lie on your back with your knees bent, feet hip width apart – gently scoop your tummy muscles in – then hug your knees into your chest one at a time. Place one hand on each knee, relax your shoulders, breathe in through your nose and out through your mouth, relax into the stretch. Enjoy 5 breaths in and out.

Beverley Densham www.mindfulnesspilates.com

Good, old-fashioned household remedies

One of the wonderful benefits of ditching the booze is that you really start to take responsibility for your own health and wellbeing in a way that you didn't before.

The old drinking you might have been regularly popping pills for every ailment; the new, conscious you will be starting to see the important correlation between what you consume (or don't), the importance of your mindset, and how your mind can literally heal your body. You will also hopefully have a sense of just how essential it is to get out in nature and practise good self-care. It's a topic I have written about extensively in my other books, so if you are interested check out the reading list and some of the recommendations, but I really hope that you will be darkening the door of the pharmacist far less often, and perhaps have fewer trips to the GP too.

Here's a quick guide to a few holistic suggestions for common ailments that can be treated, at least initially, using old-fashioned, kitchen cupboard remedies. Once again, I remind you, I'm not a doctor, and that these are just simple tips which have worked for me in the past. In every case (unless you happen to be highly allergic to a specific food or plant-based remedy), they can do no harm. You can find plenty more of these on my website or in my books.

- **Hay fever**

  Honey – do you know the honey theory? Start taking local honey to desensitise yourself to local pollens as early as possible, around February. I'm sure you know the usual stuff, too, about covering up and using a protective barrier such as the Haymax balm found in health shops (or at www.haymax.biz). The other thing that works a treat for hay fever is regular ginger shots.

- **Headaches**

  I've met many people who find the headaches that have bothered them for years just stop coming once alcohol is out of the picture, but in the first few weeks, headaches can be common – obviously from withdrawal. Drink copious amounts of water – sounds too simple but it really helps! Herbal teas are great too, tryvalerian tea, ginger tea, peppermint tea and chamomile tea which in particular is said to work in a similar way to the homeopathic remedy Feverfew, which homeopaths sometimes prescribe for headaches. If you have been used to taking aspirin, you may know that it's based on the natural remedy Willowbark, and you can buy this in health food stores.

  One of the best ways to relieve a headache is to apply gentle pressure. Either get someone else to give you a gentle head massage or do it yourself using tiny circular movements around the temples and around the eyes, and with tiny pinching movements around the jaw line. You can apply a tiny amount of the balm, you will have heard of Tiger Balm, but for a balm that is free from petrochemicals it's always best to make your own essential balm. A couple of drops of peppermint essential oil in carrier oil work well, especially to help clear the sinuses. Remember, in days of old, people who felt faint were offered lavender bags, so definitely use fresh lavender if you have it, or put a few drops of lavender or ginger essential oil on a cotton pad and breathe it in.

- **Period pains**
  It took me a good number of years before I realised that eating copious amounts of chocolate and drinking wine was not, in fact, helpful for period cramps or pre-menstrual tension. When women get more in tune with their cycle, rest when needed, and nurture themselves with good food and self-care, they can find period problems lesson. It's worth getting some professional advice if this is an area where you suffer: see a herbalist, naturopath or homeopath if you can, who may recommend herbs such as Belladonna 30C, Mag Phos and Agnus Castus for heavy periods. Most people have heard of using evening primrose oil too, and early nights with a hot water bottle can be very comforting.

- **Upset stomach**
  You know what I am going to say! Once you have ditched the booze, upset stomachs are a rare thing. I lost track of the times I had digestive issues, stomach pains and vomiting – and I always put it down to a fragile constitution and poor digestive health. I just needed to stop poisoning myself!

  If you are unlucky enough to have an upset stomach and you suspect it's nothing too serious – just something you ate, or a minor bug – let nature take its course. Fast for a day and just have plenty of fluids. Fresh mint tea is great as is peppermint and chamomile.

Skincare

As well as looking at what we put into our body, we should also look at what we put on our body. Is your skincare making you sick?

You may be wondering what this has to do with ditching the booze and focusing on optimum health and wellbeing. A lot, actually. Our skin is our largest organ and what we put on our skin, goes within. I'm sure you have heard the phrase, 'Don't put anything on your skin that you can't eat.' I wouldn't especially want to eat my mineral foundation or my lippy, but if I had to I would be fine.

The great news is that, after a possible initial period of breakouts when we ditch the booze, most women tend to find their skin clears, and they literally glow. This is because we are no longer dehydrating ourselves or putting in too many toxins.

The problem, of course, is that ditching the booze is just one part of this. What we eat and environmental toxins will all have an effect – and if you are still using conventional cosmetics and skincare, you are putting an unnecessary burden on your body and just increasing the toxic load.

There are literally thousands of synthetic chemicals passed safe for use in cosmetics, but no one has calculated what happens when they interact, so don't assume that just because it's sold on the high street, your highly perfumed cream or the cheap shampoo won't cause irritation and worse. Of course, it's not the one bottle of anything that will do any harm, it's the cumulative effects of the hundreds of different chemicals the average women has in her home, whether that's in the bathroom cabinet, in her makeup bag, or under the sink for cleaning the home.

Once we ditch the booze, we do tend to start to care more about what we consume. If we are no longer consuming alcohol and other potentially harmful chemicals, why would we want them on our skin?

I'd love to remind you that there is a natural alternative to everything. Just as you don't have to deprive yourself of a nice drink because you have chosen not to drink alcohol, so you don't need to go bare-faced or smell anything less than sweet because you have decided to ditch the chemicals too.

The bottom line is, we all use too many products. You can simplify this, save money and help the environment. You can easily make your own skincare products too, it's quick and simple.

Buy some raw extra virgin coconut oil and ensure that you have some essential oils such as lavender. Remember that coconut oil is liquid at a high temperature but then solidifies when it's cold, so keep a long-handled spoon by the jar in the bathroom for when it looks like white lard! You just need a dollop the size of a ten-pence piece, and it will turn to oil as your rub your hands together. Use it as you would any other body oil, and if you want to add a drop or two of lavender oil, go ahead. Interestingly you will find that the raw coconut oil doesn't really smell of anything. If you are expecting that strong coconut smell you experience in sun products, you're thinking of the synthetic product which has probably never seen a fresh coconut!

Coconut oil also makes a fantastic hair conditioner. If you aren't planning a night of passion, wash your hair, then apply coconut oil and wrap in a towel. While you are at it, put some on your hands and feet and wear gloves and socks. In the morning, wash it all off and voilà – silky soft.

There are a few kitchen cupboard ingredients that will be your friends for skincare. A handful of oatmeal with a bit of water makes a gentle facial wash, and adding sea salt creates an exfoliating scrub. Honey is wonderful to add to a mix of coconut oil and oatmeal, and raw cacao powder mixed with coconut oil makes an indulgent antioxidant face mask.

When you buy products, opt for the natural sustainable alternatives. There is a wealth of choice, but be careful of greenwashing and marketing spin. The word *organic* doesn't actually mean very much, it can be used in a brand name to imply that a product is 'natural' – but just because something contains 0.2 per cent organic aloe vera, for example, does not make it a natural product! Of course, if skincare is close to 100 per cent organic, then you are onto a winner.

In short, when you are buying skincare and cosmetics, look for what's *not* in the product rather than what is. Chamomile shampoo may sound lovely, but not if it contains a whole host of chemicals and just a bit of the chamomile!

The ingredients to avoid include parabens, sodium laurel sulphate, formaldehyde, perfume (be careful, this can also be listed as parfum or fragrance), phthalates, alcohol (obv), isopropyl and petroleum and mineral oil-based products.

For an extensive list of what to avoid and how to navigate cosmetics, check out the Environmental Working Group: www.ewg.org

Forget the Botox! Regular holistic facials can be one of the best ways to ensure that your skin looks toned and plumped. A good facial massage using nontoxic ingredients can help with blood flow and the lymphatic system, as well as helping us to feel calm. Facial reflexology can be amazing too. Just be sure that your therapist doesn't reach behind the couch and use synthetic creams!

Using a facial restoring tool has become my absolute favourite skincare routine. I was introduced to Gua Sha by Katie Brindle, creator of the Hayo'u Method. She gave me her jade beauty restorer, a piece of jade that fits into the palm of your hand, and showed me how to massage it across my face to stimulate the dermis, which in turn supports collagen and elastin production and releases tension. It's a bit like 'combing' your face, but it feels lovely and cool, and I am convinced it has helped my skin look brighter and more radiant.

Chapter 18
THE SOBER SOUL

As I said in the final chapter of my first book *Imperfectly Natural Woman*, the most important message I want you to know is that you are already beautiful. That is, if your energy is flowing. I wrote about some of the Hollywood stars I had been lucky enough to meet working as a presenter at BBC Radio 2; about how beautiful they were, and how their sex appeal was obvious, but how they just didn't radiate beauty, or kindness or joy. By contrast, other people were not especially known for their looks, but they lit up the room. It's so important to understand that energy is not just about how much get-up-and-go we have; our energy system is the key to our wellbeing.

Caroline Shola Arewa, known as the Energy Doctor, believes that we are energy beings and can activate our core energy for health and wellbeing:

Creating abundant energy is not as difficult as it seems. Here are two simple exercises.

1. **Breathe and relax** For just two minutes, stop what you are doing, slow down and be completely mindful of your breath. This reoxygenates, rejuvenates and relaxes your body and mind. This in turn creates calm and greater clarity. If you doubt two minutes can make a difference, give this exercise a try now!

2. **Positive self-talk** Did you know that you talk to yourself more than anyone else talks to you? What do you say? Limiting beliefs and judgemental self-talk zaps energy in a big way. If the way you talk to yourself is anything other than positive and encouraging, change the script. From now on, try to always speak to yourself kindly as you would speak to a valued friend.

Core energy can be activated by introducing simple lifestyle habits that will bring happiness and success within your reach.

Caroline Shola Arewa www.energy4lifecoach.com

The power of essential oils

A wonderful way to a tune to your senses is aromatherapy. Essential oils are great to add to skincare, to use medicinally and, of course, to lift your spirits. You can burn essential oils, or add to carrier oils and massage oils. It wasn't until I interviewed author and aromatherapist Heather Dawn Godfrey for my podcast that I realised the power of essential oils, especially for use in meditation.

Heather explains its power:

A wisp of scent is enough to immediately transport us on a sensory journey – a jasmine kiss on a starlit night; a rose garden in summer; the earthy-agrestic woodiness of a northern forest in spring; Mediterranean citrus groves in winter – sunshine on the cloudiest day. Tones, colours and shades, nuances that seamlessly imbue from conjured images, memories and impressions, complex and deep, often experienced beyond words, sensually illuminated by the gift of smell.

Magical. Yet, scent detection is initially instigated by a *chemical* response.

When we smell and acknowledge the scent of a flower or a fruit, even the scent of the soft skin of a new-born infant, we are responding to messages instigated by odour molecules permeating our immediate environment. Scent molecules (terpenes and terpenoids) are detected (like a key in a lock) by olfactory receptors located at the top of each nasal cavity, [which] in turn relay nerve impulses to the Limbic System located in the brain. Odour receptors are also located in other parts of the body – for example, in the skin and other organs.

The boundaries between physical, psychological and emotional (body, mind and spirit) often overlap, and essential oils are shown to influence these both independently and together. Indeed, feeling happy, relaxed and calm, positive and optimistic demonstrably influences physical function; heart rate, blood pressure, cortisol levels, endorphin release, digestion, and so on. Therefore, our state of 'being' (that is, 'being in stress' or 'being in equanimity', 'being in fear' or 'being in peace') can have significant influence on immunological support and healthy function.

There are various ways essential oils can be safely, effectively and conveniently dispensed and applied: diffused to create a particular ambiance; blended as a perfume in a base, such as jojoba, cream or lotion; a few drops added to an aroma-stick inhaler; or even a few drops on a tissue or cotton-pad to inhale at your leisure.

Essential oils are wonderful meditation and relaxation companions (applied using any of the above methods). For example, stimulating, refreshing and invigorating, peppermint clears the sinuses, eases breathing, and dispels feelings of tiredness without being over-stimulated. Sweet marjoram is soothing to an overactive mind. Frankincense, myrrh and patchouli calm and regulate breathing, and when combined with bitter orange, lime or another citrus oil, also dispel feelings of anxiety and depression. The earthy-smoky scent of vetivert encourages feelings of tranquillity and supports withdrawal from addiction, and when combined with the rose-like scent of geranium, and a citrus, such as grapefruit, creates a grounding, reassuring yet uplifting blend. Cypress encourages us to 'walk tall' and move on, especially as we step out of winters cave or transition from a sense of feeling 'stuck'. Rose, the 'queen of oils', blesses us with a sense of beauty and rejuvenation, and lavender gifts us its calming, uplifting, and protective qualities. The list is endless. In fact, essential oils marry beautifully with any process requiring appreciation of the moment and its endless gifts: with life itself, yours to discover!

Check the therapeutic properties of an essential oil before you apply it; do not apply neat to your skin, instead dilute essential oils in an emollient, such as vegetable oil or non-perfumed cream or lotion (one drop in 2 to 3ml of your chosen carrier medium); and do not take essential oils internally.

This article includes material and research from the books *Essential Oils for Mindfulness and Meditation and Essential Oils for the Whole Body*, Heather Dawn Godfrey, www.Inner Traditions.com

Meditation

Jo De Rosa is the founder of Quantum Sobriety and believes she is literally a different person to the one she was 20 years ago. She says:

This journey has been through meditation and the rewiring of the brain. My practice is now central to my happiness, good health, success and sobriety. In meditation we take the outside layer of life off, and sit for a period of time with ourselves, who we really are. Not who we pretend to be, or would like to be, and it's actually not even who we are, rather what we are. I have always called this part of us our 'essence', but you can call it any other name that resonates.

I overcame all of my addictions, to not only come out the other side alive, but to find *freedom* in my sobriety. I have created a whole new reality for myself, one where I never wish I could have just one glass of wine with dinner or just one line of coke or cigarette. That part of me that hankered over substances has *gone*; I'm simply not that person anymore, and there is absolutely no effort on my part to be here. I am totally free.

It is *never* too late to learn how to meditate (or to stop drinking). Buddhists call a session of sitting on your cushion 'mind training', and the truth is we can tame our unruly minds with a commitment of just 15 minutes of meditation every day. We begin to get some perspective in meditation and start the process of 'letting go', for if we can learn to let go of thoughts as they pass through the mind in meditation, then we can take this quality from our 'formal' (meditation) practice to the 'informal' (rest of our life) experience.

To begin a practice, don't over-complicate it; sit quietly and focus on the breath. Train the mind to be in one place and notice the inhale and exhale, but also the gaps/spaces in between; for these are the entry points to our magical essence. The more you practise, the more you experience who/what you truly are, thus stabilising authentic peace. Regular short sessions, even just ten minutes a couple of times per day, will help you come into alignment, step off the merry-go-round of addiction, and find *freedom* in sobriety.

Sit comfortably on the floor with your legs crossed, or in a chair. Become aware of your breath, noticing without judgement the length and quality. Notice how your body feels in its sitting position, again with no judgement. Already you are becoming the observer, the watcher, and now start to watch your thoughts as they pass through your mind like clouds.

Have you noticed how clouds don't stop in the sky? They are constantly moving, sometimes fast, sometimes slow. See if you can decipher the space between you (consciousness) and your thoughts (things). Do this for however long you have to sit.

Another technique that you can try is to visualise yourself watching a movie on a large screen. The screen and the images that you see are your thoughts, but 'you' are not the images; you are the projector, the consciousness from whence the images came. In the same way as the clouds in the sky, notice the space in-between you and the screen.

Top Tips to Get Started

Meditate in the same place every day, so that you create a positive association with this area of your home

Light a candle, use essential oils or burn some incense to set the scene; this will help to 'anchor' your practice.

The time of day is very important, with first thing in the morning before you have fully woken up the absolute best time.

If your mind is very busy, you may want to listen to recorded meditations which will help train your mind. Decide how long you are going to meditate for and set a timer or choose a recorded meditation of that time. In the beginning this only needs to be five, ten or fifteen minutes; the most important aspect here is that you are creating a new habit, a new pathway in the brain. Do not force anything. Start slowly and gently and gradually build your practice up over time.

Get comfortable and then try not to move unless you have to. Sit in a chair if being on the floor cross-legged is not an option.

Your posture wants to be strong yet relaxed: sit tall with the your back straight and shoulders wide, and then let the rest of the body relax around this frame.

Breathe in *and* out through your nose.

Make sure you are not going to be disturbed. Turn your phone off, close the door and let your family know you will be back in five, ten or twenty minutes, and then take your watch off [and put it in front of you] so that you can see the time at a glance.

Finally enjoy this 'you' time. It is the most unselfish act you can make as being calmer yourself means that you bring a more peaceful attitude to every single relationship in your life…

Jo De Rosa www.quantumsobriety.com

Hypnosis

One of the easiest ways to start to get into a meditative state is by listening to a hypnosis audio meditation. If I'd been writing this 20 years ago, you might read 'hypnosis' and think 'stage hypnotism' – being 'controlled' to sit in a bath of baked beans, for example – but most people are now aware of the benefits of hypnosis for behaviour change. I had many hypnosis sessions before I had my first baby and I am convinced it helped me to overcome some of my insecurities and embrace motherhood, despite the pregnancy being an accident after I'd vowed to never have children (I know; I had four!).

In recent years I have co-authored hypnosis audio apps with one of the leading hypnosis authors, Glenn Harrold. (Our most recent is *Quit the Alcohol Habit Forever*.) Hypnosis is simply the ability to focus your attention on a specific aim, whilst in a deeply relaxed state of mind and body. Quitting alcohol or any habit can leave a vacuum, and it is important to replace those old habits with new positive, healthy routines that you actually enjoy, as that is the key to them having longevity.

After quitting booze, you can use self-hypnosis to reinforce new habits and routines and embrace a new healthy lifestyle. Glenn Harrold offers us this simple exercise:

- Close your eyes, take a few slow deep breaths in through your nose and out through your mouth. Continue this breathing motion and clear away all thought, so your mind becomes very still and quiet.
- The goal is no thought at all, and you achieve this state by letting go and surrendering, rather than forcing it. Just continue to breathe away all cares and worries with every outbreath, and allow yourself to drift ever deeper.
- Once you get to a point where you are very still and centred, imagine your new healthy lifestyle in detail. Visualise yourself free of the booze habit and immersed in new healthy activities and really enjoying this new direction. Engage your feelings and connect with positive emotions as you visualise, as this deepens the effect. Make your visualisations as colourful and detailed as possible as when you visualise in a relaxed state your mind doesn't distinguish between what is real and what is imagined. By creating colourful, detailed visualisations, you are able to create powerful new mental programmes that become anchored in your unconscious mind.

Glenn Harrold www.glennharrold.com

Using self-hypnosis will help you make the adjustment from the old to the new and by working with your unconscious mind the results will be lasting and effective. The transition from old unwanted habits to a new healthy lifestyle is an easy process when you use the full power of your mind.

The key to self-hypnosis is to remain focused on your goals, in spite of any distractions or mental chatter. If you do get distracted at any time, empty your mind and take a few deep breaths and you will naturally drift deeper again. Then refocus on your goal.

The state you are aiming to create is one of strong focus where you are deeply relaxed and your mind is calm free from thought. Using your feelings is the key part of using self-hypnosis successfully, especially when you focus on specific goals.

When you achieve deep physical relaxation with a strong mental focus *and* you are engaging your feelings, the effect will be powerful and lasting.

I asked Sober Club members to list some benefits of sobriety, what happened when their lives shifted from the old to the new. I quickly realised I could fill the whole book. I would like to share some of these with you:

Being a present parent.
Always knowing where your purse is after an evening out.
Waking up in the morning and remembering everything from the night before including going to bed.
Being able to drive anytime day or night.
No pop-up parties at my house that I invited people to without remembering I did!
Belly bloat and 13 pounds gone!
More energy.
Being able to really 'feel' my emotions.
8+ hours uninterrupted sleep per night.
Being a good role model for my family and making them proud.
Discovering new hobbies that require focused concentration.
Proper memories that I can actually remember!
Mornings...such lovely early mornings!
No arguments with husband about having a 'last' drink.

Less anxiety and not over-reacting to everything.
Sense of much-increased resilience.
Skin improvement.
I've slowed down a lot & I'm kinder to myself.
Not waking up with that 'Shit, what did I say or do?'
Mental clarity.
Zero shame and anxiety.
Self-respect.
The feeling of joy.

Joy

I think I rarely used the word *joy* before ditching booze. It seemed like something reserved for young children or happy-clappy church services, it certainly wasn't anything that grumpy old me would have experienced.

When I read Catherine Gray's *The Unexpected Joy of Being Sober*, the word really resonated with me. It was expertly chosen. The dictionary definition of *joy* is: the emotion of great delight or happiness caused by something exceptionally good or satisfying; keen pleasure; elation.

It really is that feeling of happiness, and satisfaction that is so surprising. It's the joy of everyday things, and the absolute elation that many of us have literally not experienced since we were children. This is our natural default state as humans, it's just that we have managed to dampen ourselves down and numb ourselves out so that we need to take substances to be able to artificially create a kind of fun But then the scales come off and you realise that being drunk isn't fun at all. Being fully present, alive and aware is where it's at, sometimes joyful, sometimes calm, but always conscious and stable.

Chapter 19
THE SOBER LIFESTYLE

Creativity. Where does creativity fit in?

I have heard so many people say that they found creativity when they ditched the booze. But others, especially writers, musicians and artists, fear that when they stop drinking they will lose their creative ability. Somehow being creative has been linked to being hedonistic and 'out of it'. I've known people continue to drink simply because they think they will no longer have ideas once the edge of their addiction, despair or craziness has been taken away. Creatives fear that their wild side is what makes them able to create. Once they are stable, not taking risks or behaving badly, their art will become like their life – boring!

Let me remind you again: *sober* does not equal *bores*. In fact, once you are through the tricky stage, when the brain chemistry starts to kick back in, you will hopefully be able to find even more creative ways to get your dopamine hit. Instead of taking yourself to the edge with mood-altering drugs, you will learn to choose healthy ways of seeking and receiving pleasure.

Despite popular opinion, you don't have to be traumatised to create great art or music. What you do need to be able to do is feel, really feel what's going on. Before, while you were drinking, perhaps everything was numbed. By pushing yourself a little out of your comfort zone, you may find you are creative and have some profound stories to share.

Creativity can take many forms, but before we get into art and its therapeutic effects, let's look at creative writing. As I said earlier, keeping a journal can be one of the best tools in your sober toolkit and it is like an act of kindness to yourself to get your thoughts out and onto paper. It's important to remember that the art of writing is about letting out your thoughts, to release what's bubbling around in the unconscious mind, but it's important to do it for its own sake, not for the purpose of being edited or read by others.

I was lucky enough to contribute to a writer's workshop where the main speaker was Julia Cameron, the author, artist, poet, playwright, filmmaker and composer. She is most famous for *The Artist's Way*, a book that has now sold several million copies and which remains a classic, one that should be on the bookshelf of anyone who wants to expand their creativity.

Julia is a fantastic workshop leader, giving us great insights into how to kick-start our creativity. She insists:

The bedrock tool of a creative recovery is a daily practice called Morning Pages. She believes it's imperative to write the Morning Pages. At least three pages of longhand every morning, preferably when you first wake up. I'm guessing you had to go back and re-read that – yes, I did say *longhand*, i.e. handwriting – remember that? No laptops, tablets or phones, good old-fashioned pen and paper! There's something unique about letting the words flow onto a page. Julia reminded us that there is no right way or wrong way to do it (and yes, you can have a cup of coffee), but you must write everything that comes into your head. Don't think about it, or edit, or assess, just write – and don't show them to anyone, they are only for you. Unsure what to write? Just write anyway, it's a stream of consciousness, it might include: Oops forgot to send a birthday card to Dawn…I'm feeling really excited if apprehensive about my next big speaking gig…why do I keep thinking about wine, I haven't a clue what to wear when it's this cold…I so don't want to go to the gym… You get the idea! It can be about nothing – and everything. Interestingly, the act of writing it down is very cathartic and brings peace. It's rather like a creative form of meditation, but whereas many of us find meditation difficult because we are trying *not* to have thoughts, the idea here is to download as many as possible; Julia says spirituality and creativity are intrinsically linked. If you are a writer, Julia believes you are also a critic, and she believes this simple daily practice helps you over time to choose positive attitudes. In order to let all the thoughts flow, you have to ask your critic to step aside – and let's face it in the search for perfection, many of us are literally silenced by our inner voices most of the time. I've lost count of the clients who tell me they know they should change their career, write their book, share their story, travel… live their dreams – but procrastination or fear of being judged is holding them back. Give it a shot; if you are currently trying to make some sense of your life and work, it's one of the best tools I know to fast-track you to clarity and to get those creative juices flowing. People often find other areas of their life improve when they start writing daily.

Check out her website: www.juliacameronlive.com

'Seeing ourselves' – sobriety and art

Sharon Walters is an artist who creates hand-assembled collages celebrating Black women. The series 'Seeing Ourselves' explores under-representation in the Arts and Heritage sector and in Western media. Her work encourages us to 'take up space and be seen', and I asked her to share a bit of her story:

> I came across some old magazines, a cutting mat and some glue from when I had made collages. I started to flick through the magazines and became intrigued by the lack of Black women who looked back at me from the pages. Every time I saw one, I would cut the photo out and create a portrait collage. I wanted the work to talk about nature, Afro hair and beauty standards. I wanted to readdress the balance and the lack of representation of Black women in many arenas, including arts and heritage, particularly of interest as I worked in a museum and rarely saw others like me.

I always thought I did not have time to create, but I realise now this theory was not entirely true. My time was allocated elsewhere, and my aspirations had been obscured by alcohol. Now two and half years into the series and a year and a half sober, I have had many exhibitions, sold my work globally, spoken about sobriety and creativity on panels and delivered collage and sobriety workshops, and have over 250 collages in the 'Seeing Ourselves' collection. I certainly have not got more time than I had prior to sobriety, how I choose to spend my time has changed.

I now create collages almost daily and enter a space where my mind is at rest, I get to a point where the work just flows. The process of trusting intuition, removing sections through collage to create something new is reminiscent of my ideas around removing alcohol from my life. I was unsure of the outcome, but it has created a beautiful and unimaginable life.

My advice to anyone who would like to get started is to dedicate ten minutes a day to being creative. It is important to trust the process rather than the outcome. The focus should be on how the creative practice makes you feel. We are so often our own worst critics, but this can also mean we end up 'standing in our own way', which can leave us immobile and afraid to try new things or return to childhood ambitions.

Art has become a part of my therapy. It continues to help me through sobriety, soothing me, a replacement for a 'cheeky glass of wine'. There is, of course, the reality of the danger in handling a cutting knife while drinking, but I no longer feel the need to numb feelings or 'celebrate' with alcohol. I now give myself permission to 'feel' all the emotions, not always welcome, but I appreciate the joys in what I have achieved through sobriety. I have a long way to go and many dreams still to achieve, but I now see these are possible.

Sharon Walters www.londonartist1.com

Sober firsts and holidays

Your first year sober is a year of firsts, and they are all rather like climbing mountains: they feel utterly huge and overwhelming, but once you are at the top, it's all good and you wonder what the fuss was about. Within the first few months of sobriety, most people have to prepare for and experience their first social occasion, work event, family gathering (party, wedding or christening) and, of course, their first holiday. Holidays are so associated with drinking, it's actually ludicrous. We all know how time stands still at airports, so of course it's fine to drink at 7 a.m., and why not drink champagne throughout the flight? It would be rude not to. For me flying was intrinsically linked with drinking, and I must confess I was nervous before I took my first flight. Fortunately, it was a morning flight to Scotland, so I didn't feel any pressure to drink, but even then the person in the seat next to me was knocking back Vodka and Tonics like they were going out of fashion.

If your idea of a holiday is a cruise or an all-inclusive, there is the added pressure of feeling that you have paid for the booze, so you are going to be seriously missing out. There have been many people who cave in on holiday because they want to join in with their family and friends and feel relaxed and there are simply no options other than water available. But is that true now? Absolutely not. As with everything, your key to staying sober through your first sober holiday and beyond is to prep ahead. If you are packing a suitcase, stash it with alcohol-free drinks of your choice. If it's an all-inclusive ring the hotel (or cruise ship) ahead of time and state your dietary requirements, just as you would if you were vegan. You can ask for some decent grown up alcohol-free drinks, i.e. *not* soft drinks, but good alcohol-free beers, and mocktails. Make friends with the bartenders and you will usually be OK. If push comes to shove, take your own little bottles of botanical alternatives to spirits and order a tonic water pimped with everything – ask for a G&T without the G.

I did my first all-inclusive, and it was actually a breeze. I took a bottle of alcohol-free wine, but the bar made me virgin mojitos. The first one was super sweet, but I asked for less syrup after that.

This holiday I enjoyed more than any other. I was up by 6.30 a.m. every day (commandeering the sunbeds) and enjoying lovely beach walks on my own before everyone surfaced.

Always try to book yourself into activities early in a morning, even if you are only on a short weekend break. It's the key to ensuring that you won't give in late at night, because you have something the next day that you want to be fresh for.

There are sober holiday and retreats and mindful drinking festivals in London and these kinds of events will grow. Check the resources section and if there is nothing near where you live, consider starting something! Don't forget The Sober Club!

If you are looking for a sober break, I offer *Self-care in Sobriety* retreats and there are wonderful solo holidays (see resources for recommendations).

How are your ZZZs?

When I stopped drinking, I fully expected to be sleeping like a baby within a few days. I had read about the lovely deep sleep and waking refreshed that sober people talked about.

I got a bit of a shock to find that my sleep was wholly disrupted. I'd find myself lying awake anxious and fearful, I'd have weird dreams and even leg cramps (magnesium deficiency perhaps), and occasionally I'd get panicky thoughts about drinking. I'd wake with a start, convinced I had turned back to drink. I've since found out it is very common to have drinking dreams, but they sure scare you when you get them!

Issues with sleep are not confined to people ditching the booze, of course; some claim there is a nationwide deficiency of sleep. Not getting enough, or enough good quality sleep, is so detrimental to our health and wellbeing.

Alcohol and good sleep are not good bedfellows, that's for sure. Drinking can disrupt your sleep cycles so that we feel sluggish and tired during the day, and in turn that affects our mood.

There is the misconception that alcohol helps us to sleep, but while alcohol can indeed cause you to pass out fairly quickly, we will then not spend enough time in the important REM (rapid eye movement) sleep, which is the important restorative stage that we need.

Obviously alcohol is a diuretic too, so you may find you need the loo during the night – how many people put that down to old age? Many people wake up feeling dehydrated. If you sleep with someone who drinks a lot of alcohol, you may have noticed that they snore loudly too; that's because alcohol can relax the muscles so the air doesn't flow smoothly.

If you are in the early stages and sleep is eluding you, I can only dangle that carrot on a stick and tell you that once it comes (for me it was after about 3–4 weeks) sober sleep is incredible. It's *so* different because you get proper quality sleep, and when you wake, instead of that awful shaky feeling of trying out one eye, checking whether you are hungover, or indeed in your own bed, you wake feeling refreshed and content. The first time it happened to me, I couldn't quite place the feeling. I lay there in a fuzzy state and thought: *What's that feeling?*. I realised with amazement that it was contentment.

If you haven't tried sobriety yet, am I persuading you? Trust me, it's worth it for the sleep alone!

So, what can we do while we wait? Well, yet again nutrition plays its part. It's well worth ensuring that you have good protein levels and some tryptophan before bed. Try warm drinks such as herbal tea – chamomile is great – and you can try the Sing Me to Sleep tea from Chuckling Goat. You may also have heard of 'sleep hygiene'. This is the basics, essentially: sleep in a dark room, get blackout curtains if you need them, get your electronic devices out of the bedroom, turn off the Wi-Fi if possible, and ensure that you have a comfortable mattress and pillows.

This next one is important. Turn off from all screens at least an hour before you go to sleep. This is key, we are meant to have a 'sundown', a time to wind down, so most definitely do *not* watch the late TV news!

One nutritionist I interviewed, Heather Nickel, believes we should go to bed by 10 p.m. Ouch! How will I get everything done? That may not work for you, but do remember the old saying: the more hours before midnight, the better.

There are some well-known tips for good sleep:

- Having a warm bath with essential oils can be very relaxing. Add some magnesium or Epsom salts, and you can also add a blob of organic coconut oil (saves you needing to put moisturiser on afterwards!). You can also drop some Lavender oil on your pillow or burn some in a diffuser.

- Check out the herbal remedies for sleep too. Valerian is well known, but there is also a supplement called Asphalia, which was originally produced to help with electromagnetic pollution, but is also said to aid good sleep. You can also get homeopathic drops that help with sleep; try Weleda's sleep remedy, Avena Sative.

- Clear your mind, this can be the single best tip. Write down ten things that you are grateful for, and put them down in detail. So rather than just 'I'm grateful for my home', flesh out the detail – why? Were there interactions during the day that you are grateful for?

- You may want to ensure that you have written a priority list for the next day. Preferably do that before you head to bed, so that you don't lie there stressing about what you might forget the next day.

- Work with your dreams. When we sleep, our unconscious mind is sorting everything out for us and making sense of it all. If you recall a dream, jot it down (always have a notebook and pen by the bed). You might want to analyse what it's telling you.

Robyn Spens is a hypnotherapist and functional nutrition practitioner who offers the following advice:

> Sleep rejuvenates our brain and our body, consolidates our memory, detoxes our brain and processes emotion. Outside of a genuine sleep disorder such as sleep apnoea and narcolepsy, lack of sleep is mainly a stress and lifestyle management issue.
>
> Not getting the required amount can affect your health in a variety of ways from hormone disruption, obesity, higher

risk of heart disease [and] dementia and for some, lack of sleep presents safety issues at work. The National Sleep Foundation suggests we need between 7 and 9 hours of sleep each night. It seems very few of us are adhering to this advice.

While there are various natural solutions to tackle insomnia and sleep disorders, alcohol and sleeping tablets are not. They cause dependency and a whole host of other problems. More natural recommendations include eating probiotic rich foods, valerian tea, passion flower, magnesium and melatonin – which should be used minimally as it down-regulates your natural production. Before choosing I suggest you seek clarification and guidance from your GP or health specialist regarding their suitability.

What makes a good sleep protocol?

- Start the wind down process when the sun goes down
- Relax the brain before bed with meditation
- Listen to hypnosis recording or learn self-hypnosis
- Reduce light in the bedroom
- Reduce the heating in the bedroom
- Remove the TV and computer to reduce exposure to blue light before bed
- Go to bed and get up at the same time
- Expose your eyes to light first thing in the morning to raise cortisol levels and lower melatonin
- Don't eat meals after 8 p.m.

Robyn Spens www.robynspens.com

Yoga Nidra

Years ago, I was on a juice detox retreat. One day, I'd done two yoga classes and a fair bit of exercise, and when the yoga guru asked us all to reconvene for Yoga Nidra at 8 p.m. I was thinking of giving it a miss. He saw the look on my face and explained that Yoga Nidra requires no movement whatsoever; it's the yoga of sleep, literally just relaxation. I got into comfortable clothes, took my yoga mat and duvet out to the deck and experienced the most amazing relaxation. It was a wonderful introduction to Yoga Nidra. I have since recorded my own Yoga Nidra chakra meditation called The Yoga of Sleep. It's thought that an hour of Yoga Nidra is equivalent to about four hours sleep, so it's a wonderful way to get your ZZZs.

Dealing with stress

Anxiety, stress, panic – we have all been there. As I've already said, I didn't really appreciate just how manic and anxious I was until I got sober and started to feel a sense of equilibrium. There was often still stress in my life, but I felt more resilient, more able to deal with it. I remember when I was just over three months sober, I had my purse stolen from my bag while I was out having coffee. I was in a blind panic for a few moments, frantically asking people in the coffee shop, calling my husband because I simply couldn't remember what I needed to do under severe stress. After just a few moments I took a breath, and realised that yes, it was an inconvenience – I had lost a fair bit of cash, all my credit cards and a few important numbers written on paper stored in my wallet – but I hadn't lost my phone or my keys. I was on the way to a yoga class, and realised I would need to go into the bank and cancel my main debit card, so I rang the gym and said I would be a few minutes late but could I still attend? They were lovely and said yes. It was the most perfect antidote to that stress. I counted my blessings and then went to yoga and relaxed. I don't think I would have been that calm if I had been drinking. The 'poor me' mentality would have continued for way longer, and I'd have been weeping and wailing, certainly not in the frame of mind for a yoga class!

That's one example, but there were and still are literally loads of times when I feel as though my to-do list is endless, I have too many deadlines fast approaching and I find myself saying: 'I feel stressed!'

But what is stress really, and how does it affect us? I asked Neil Shah, bestselling author, entrepreneur and CEO of Stress Management Society and two years sober. He and his team are dedicated to leading effective universal change by maximising resilience, happiness, productivity and success with their passionate approach to reducing stress and promoting wellbeing. Neil says:

Firstly, let's debunk one myth: stress is not necessarily a 'bad' thing. Without this brilliant ability to experience stress, humankind wouldn't have survived. Our cavemen ancestors, for example, used the onset of stress to alert them to a potential danger, such as a sabre-toothed tiger. Through the release of hormones such as adrenaline, cortisol and norepinephrine, the caveman gained a rush of energy, which prepared him to either fight the tiger or run away. That heart pounding, fast breathing sensation is the adrenaline; as well as a boost of energy, it enables us to focus our attention so we can quickly respond to the situation.

In the modern world, the 'fight or flight' mode can still help us survive dangerous situations – for example, reacting swiftly to a person running in front of our car by slamming on the brakes.

The challenge is when our body goes into a state of stress in inappropriate situations. When blood flow is going only to the most important muscles needed to fight or flee, brain function is minimised. This can lead to an inability to 'think straight'; a state that is a great hindrance in both our work and home lives. If we are kept in a state of stress for long periods, it can be detrimental to our health. The results of having elevated cortisol levels can be an increase in sugar and blood pressure levels, and a decrease in libido.

A useful analogy to explain stress is that of a bridge. When a bridge is carrying too much weight, it will eventually collapse. However, before this happens it is possible to see the warning signs, such as bowing, buckling or creaking. The same principle can be applied to human beings. It is usually possible to spot early warning signs of excessive pressure that could lead to breakdown.

That 'bridge collapse' in a human being can take many forms:

- Mental and emotional breakdown
- Taking one's own life
- Serious health issues

The key message is that if we are able to recognise when we have too much demand on our bridge then we can take action to prevent ourselves from getting anywhere near the bridge collapsing, which thankfully most of us will never experience or see.

Some signs of a bowing and buckling bridge to look out for:

- Being more accident-prone
- Forgetting things
- Showing a negative change in mood or fluctuations in mood
- Avoiding certain situations or people
- Using more negative or cynical language
- Becoming withdrawn
- Showing a prolonged loss of sense of humour
- Becoming increasingly irritable or short-tempered
- Having more arguments and disputes
- A tendency to suffer from headaches, nausea, aches and pains, tiredness and poor sleeping patterns
- Indecisiveness and poor judgement
- A problem with drinking or drug taking
- Looking haggard or exhausted all the time

Things you can do to help yourself:

Get enough sleep
Work off stress with physical activity
Breathe – breathing exercises really help calm you down
And most importantly – avoid nicotine, alcohol, caffeine and refined sugar products They are all stimulants, which prevent you from feeling calm.

Neil Shah www.stress.org.uk

Anxiety and time management

One of the great benefits of ditching the booze is seeing how your anxiety levels are affected. Most people report a definite change for the better within a few days and a real noticeable change after a few weeks.

Karla McLaren, author of *Embracing Anxiety: How to Access the Genius of This Vital Emotion*, says that all our emotions have a specific purpose and brings a unique set of gifts skills and genius. She says that rather than try to make them go away (we are all taught that emotions such as sadness, anxiety, etc are bad and must seek pleasure quickly and try and get away from them) we should see them as our support system and learn to work with them.

If you started drinking at a relatively young age, you probably didn't get to experience many of life's big emotional situations sober! We were so accustomed to feeling sad, angry, fearful, and anxious – and then just numbing it with alcohol.

Anxiety, while challenging, is an essential emotion with an important job to do. It helps us to look ahead, organise ourselves and gather the energy we need to get things done.

Of course, it can get out of hand and run away with us till we feel out of control and overwhelmed. But what if it's trying to help us?

When we ignore or repress our anxiety, it can overwhelm us. But when we learn to welcome it with skill, we can access its remarkable gifts.

When you feel anxious, Karla suggests, ask yourself: 'What's bringing this emotion forward? What needs to be done?'

Sometimes it's down to finding the focus, planning, making lists, gathering the resources we need and harnessing the energy we need to complete tasks.

According to Karla, **anxiety is the 'task-completion expert of our psyche'.** It was a bit of a lightbulb moment for me when I read that anxiety often means focus, planning and concentration. That's helped me to really notice why I am feeling anxious, and usually it does mean there is a bunch of tasks I have been putting off, and if I just get on with them I will feel better. Simples, yet so often we carry on getting stressed and frustrated, procrastinating and feeling sorry for ourselves.

Karla McLaren www.karlamclaren.com

Time management

So, much of our anxiety and feelings of overwhelm come from not managing our time effectively. When we are drinking, we have so many excuses for all the lost hours (the amount of time lost to hangovers is quite incredible) and as for getting on with hobbies etc, most drinkers have stopped doing the things they used to enjoy because drinking takes up all their free hours.

So when the booze goes, there can be lots of time to fill, and rather than wandering around hoping to find some chores, set yourself a plan and track how you spend your time and what you actually want.

I began using a technique called 'Clean set-up' every morning.

I asked myself three questions:

1. *What do I want from today* (or a specific project or event)?
2. *How do I have to be for that to happen?* This is a great question because it means you have to take responsibility for your mood and actions.
3. *What resources/help do I need?* This is where you may need to structure your time, ask colleagues or family members for support or research something that will help you.

It also helps to ask yourself: *What can I do today that improves my life, my health, my wellbeing?*

Finding your purpose

Often when the booze has gone, something quite magical will happen. You discover you gain more clarity on what you really want in your life.

Sobriety is amazing at revealing truths. The truths about your job, your relationships, your life.

Sometimes you have to clear space before you can start to build the life you want. That could mean decluttering. It's very common for newly sober people to have very clean and organised homes because they get really good at decluttering! Personally I am not a Marie Kondo type of gal (I just can't roll a jumper and I really do have way too many clothes that 'spark joy'), but the theory of clearing out is a good one. It may be that in order to fulfil your purpose and live your best life you need to declutter some friends from your life too. That may sound harsh, but if you are spending valuable time with the wrong people who actually drain your energy this won't be serving you, or getting you closer to doing what you are here to do.

Choose your company, choose your tribe.

My journey started 3 July 2019. It was a night just like any other spent swilling cider at my local pub. I had convinced myself over the years that my drinking was acceptable, I surrounded myself with likeminded others and I would despise anyone who questioned my habit. But it had taken its toll on me. There was no rock bottom moment, just a slow realisation that drinking alcohol had never served me well and was responsible for the situation I found myself in.

My health was really concerning me. I had just hit a whopping 25 stone. Also I was seriously depressed with absolutely no hope for the future. Added to that, my finances were being stretched to the point I couldn't fulfil my commitments. It was at this moment I observed the people around me all in different stages of intoxication and I got a future vision of myself which I didn't like.

I made a decision there and then never to take another drink. I educated myself about alcohol addiction. I read books listened to podcasts and watched documentaries on YouTube and just concentrated on getting through one day at a time.

I started seeing the benefits almost immediately. My weight fell off, my finances improved rapidly, I started to get a more positive better outlook on life. I slept well, I rediscovered my hobbies and made new friends in a different social circle, and then before I knew it, it occurred to me that my new life was far more enjoyable than my previous drunken existence.

Roll on a year I have achieved so much. I've lost 6 stone in weight, I've started a side business which has enabled me to claw myself back financially. I have so many new interests and friends.

Sobriety has given me a peace of mind permanently whereas alcohol supplied it for tiny snippets of time followed by the inevitable comedown. It gives me everything alcohol promised but never delivered.

John Drage

Celebs and sobriety

It wasn't many years back when we all wanted our celebrities and rock stars to be badly behaved. It seemed entirely reasonable for anyone who is creative and glamourous to be on a path to destruction and it was seen to be cool to be wild, and addicted to drugs and alcohol.

There are so many sober celebrities now, it's hard to keep track, and there is something really quite comforting in knowing that we aren't alone in our struggles, even the rich and famous have their moments and live to come through to health and happiness. Somehow it validates the coolness of sobriety when we see the company we are in. It certainly encourages brands and bars and clubs to ensure they have a good stock of alcohol-free drinks. Who would want to be hosting a function where Russell Brand, Zoe Ball, Elton John arrive, and you have only red or white wine or a warm orange juice on offer!

If you want to feel inspired, do some research on Sober Celebs and know that you are in good company.

What I love is reading about how much sobriety means to them. In his autobiography, Elton John makes it clear that getting sober saved him, and he then went on to inspire so many other celebrities, including Enimen, Donatella Versace, Robbie Williams and Rufus Wainwright. Russell Brand (one of the few celebs I have actually gone a bit weak at the knees when meeting) was always known for his partying and misbehaviour, but he has written the book *Recovery*, and hosts courses on his version of the 12 Step Programme.

Here's a list of a few who have spoken publicly about their sobriety, but there are many more!

Zoe Ball, Kim Kardashian, Demi Lovata, Russell Brand, Bradley Cooper , Samuel L Jackson, Brad Pitt, Kelly Osbourne, Denise Welch, Nicole Richie, Daniel Radcliffe, Zac Efron, Rob Lowe, Jamie Lee Curtis, Kristin Davis, Gerard Butler, Edie Falco.

The times they are a-changing!

Afterword
BE A ROCKING SOBER BADASS!

I hope beyond hope that you have come to the end of this book feeling inspired, believing that it is entirely within your grasp to feel fully alive and whole, happy, full of energy and vitality. If you haven't yet quit the alcohol habit, I hope you will give it a shot, for at least 30 days, preferably longer. While you are going through the hard bit, get connected, get support, nurture yourself and be self-kind. I hope this book has dangled the carrot on the end of the stick for you to see that this is *so* worth it!

Don't let FOMO get in the way. As the title of Laura McKowen's fabulous book says: 'We are the luckiest'. I hope you feel inspired to come and be part of our gang, the rocking sober badasses who live their lives to the full.

Sobriety literally makes you brave, while alcohol steals your joy, so you have everything to look forward to, and nothing, nothing at all to lose.

I did wonder if, once I got to a year sober, I'd have experienced all the firsts and so might feel a bit flat. After the novelty of being sober had worn off, might I just hit the f— it button and decide to drink again? But I could never have imagined just how much better year on year sobriety gets. There are so many benefits that don't reveal themselves till much later down the line. You are just going to have to trust me on that one.

Sobriety is the gift that keeps on giving. I hate that phrase, it's so naff, but I can't think of a better one. As Catherine Gray said recently, 'Getting sober was the hardest, but the most beautiful thing I have ever done'.

If you have been sober for a while, I really hope this book has inspired you to take a holistic approach to other areas of your life. This is the perfect time to look at nutrition, ditching the chemicals from your life, improving your environment. It's the time to reassess your purpose, your relationships and of course your mindset.

It may be that you have discovered new things about yourself, but you need to put boundaries in place to protect who you really are.

My relentless enthusiasm and passion for sobriety doesn't mean, by the way, that I can't see how difficult it is for some people. You may have been round the block many times, but that's no reason to give up. Just try a different approach. It matters not one jot to me how you get sober. If AA meetings work for you, fantastic; if you need medication, go for it; if you connect with an online group that's great. Do whatever it takes to get free from this addictive substance and get back to the real you. You're worth it.

I do believe anyone can do it. The hard bit isn't stopping drinking, it's staying alcohol-free – and if you have done that or you are well on the way, a high five to you! We are Sober Heroes, we truly are. To be free from this addictive emotional crutch is life-changing and liberating.

If you are struggling, always ask for help. People tend to think it's a sign of weakness to ask, but the truth is by asking others you are allowing them to know it's OK to ask too! It's scientifically proven that by acts of kindness (offering help or support to others) is good for you. In fact as the giver, you receive even more than the recipient, so *ask* for help!

Elton John celebrated 30 years of being sober recently and told his 11 million followers on social media: 'If I hadn't finally taken the big step of asking for help 30 years ago, I'd be dead.' He talked about the significance of celebrating being sober for three decades, and posted a series of photographs showing anniversary cards, sobriety chips, and even a cake in the shape of a 30. 'Reflecting on the most magical day having celebrated my 30th Sobriety Birthday,' he wrote.

Isn't it amazing that it's still such a thing for him after 30 years! If you have been a drinker, choosing to be alcohol-free is not just another fad, or dietary preference. It's literally a life-changing decision that affects everything.

Always celebrate your Soberversaries; they may come to mean more to you than your birthday because that's when you really started living.

Do consider joining The Sober Club. I love hearing your stories! Please connect with me on social media @janeyleegrace

www.happyhealthysober.com

BIBLIOGRAPHY AND RECOMMENDED READING

Books

Brand, Russell *Recovery: Freedom from our Addictions* (Bluebird, 2018)

Cameron, Julia *The Artist's Way: A Spiritual Path to Higher Creativity* (Souvenir Press, 2020)

Carr, Allen *The Easy Way to Control Alcohol* (Arcturus, 2009)

Carr, Allen *The Easy Way for Women to Stop Drinking* (Arcturus, 2016)

Chapple, Simon *How to Quit alcohol in 50 days: Stop Drinking and Find Freedom* (Sheldon Press, 2020)

Dann, Lotta *Mrs D is Going Without: A Memoir* (Allen and Unwin, 2018)

De Rosa, Jo *Quantum Sobriety* (Quantum Superpowers Publishing, 2018)

Glenn, Harrold *De-stress Your Life: A new approach to reducing stress in your everyday life* (Orion Spring, 2019)

Godfrey, Heather Dawn *Essential Oils for Mindfulness and Meditation: Relax, replenish and Rejuvenate* (Healing Arts Press, 2018)

Godfrey, Heather Dawn *Essential Oils for the Whole Body: The Dynamics of Topical Application and Absorption* (Healing Arts Press, 2019)

Gooch, Millie *The Sober Girl Society Handbook: An empowering guide to living hangover free* (Bantam Press, 2021)

Grace, Annie *This Naked Mind* (Harper Collins, 2018)

Grace, Janey Lee *Imperfectly Natural Woman: Getting Life Right the Natural Way* (Crown House, 2005)

Grace, Janey Lee *Imperfectly Natural Baby and Toddler: How to be a green parent in today's busy world* (Orion, 2007)

Grace, Janey Lee *Imperfectly Natural Home: Everything you need to know to create a healthy, natural home: The Organic Bible* (Orion, 2008)

Grace, Janey Lee *Look Great Naturally ... without Ditching the Lipstick* (Hay House, 2013)

Grace, Janey Lee *You are the Brand – PR Secrets to Fastrack your Visibility and Sky-rocket your Success* (Filament Publishing, 2015)

Gray, Catherine *The Unexpected Joy of Being Sober: Discovering a happy, healthy, wealthy alcohol-free life* (Aster, 2017)

Gray, Catherine *The Unexpected joy of Being Single* (Aster, 2018)

Haidt, Jonathan *The Happiness Hypothesis: Putting Ancient Wisdom to the Test of Modern Science* (Arrow, 2007)

Hamilton, David *I Heart Me: The Science of Self-Love* (Hay House, 2015)

Hamilton, David *Why Kindness is good for you* (Hay House, 2010)

Hepola, Sarah *Blackout: Remembering the things I drank to forget* (Two Roads, 2016)

Hobson, Rob *The Art of Sleeping: the secret to sleeping better at night for a happier, calmer more successful day* (HQ, 2019)

Khechara, Star *The Holistic Beauty Book: With Over 100 Natural Recipes for Beautiful Skin* (Green Books, 2008)

Libaire, Jardine and Ward, Amanda Eyre *The Sober Lush: A Hedonist's Guide to Living a Decadent, Adventurous, Soulful Life – Alcohol Free* (Penguin Random House, 2020)

Liptrot, Amy *The Outrun* (Canongate, 2015)

Manners, Mandy and Baily, Kate *Love Yourself Sober: A Self Care Guide to Alcohol-Free Living for Busy Mothers* (Trigger Publishing, 2020)

McKowen, Laura *We are the Luckiest: The Surprising Magic of a Sober Life* (New World Library, 2020)

McLaren, Karla *Embracing Anxiety: How to Access the Genius of This Vital Emotion* (Sounds True, 2020)

Nix-Jones, Shann *The Kefir Solution: Natural Healing for IBS, Depression and Anxiety* (Hay House, 2018)

Northrup, Christiane *Goddesses Never Age: The Secret Prescription for Radiance, Vitality and Wellbeing* (Hay House, 2015)

Pooley, Clare *The Sober Diaries: How one woman stopped drinking and started living* (Coronet, 2018)

Porter, William *Alcohol Explained* (CreateSpace, 2015)

Porter, William *Alcohol Explained 2* (Independently published, 2019)

Porter, William *Diet and Fitness Explained* (Independently published, 2018)

Ramage, Andy and Fairbairns, Ruari *The 28 Day Alcohol Free Challenge: Sleep Better, Lose Weight, Boost Energy, Beat Anxiety* (Bluebird, 2017)

Roberts, Ciara Jean *Wholly Aligned, Wholly Alive: Awakening your Inner Physician* (Filament, 2019)

Rocca, Lucy *Glass Half Full: A Positive Journey to Living Alcohol-Free* (Headline Accent, 2014)

Ross, Julia *The Mood Cure: Take Charge of Your Emotions in 24 Hours Using Food and Supplements* (Thorsons, 2009)

Ross, Julia *The Diet Cure: The 8-Step Program to Rebalance Your Body Chemistry and End Food Cravings, Weight Gain, and Mood Swings--Naturally* (Penguin Random House, 2012)

Ross, Julia *The Craving Cure: Identify Your Craving Type to Activate Your Natural Appetite Control* (Flatiron Books, 2018)

Sigman, Aric *Alcohol Nation: How to protect our children from today's drinking culture* (Piatkus, 2011)

Sigman, Aric *Body Wars: Why Body Dissatisfaction is at Epidemic Proportions and How We Can Fight Back* (Piatkus, 2014)

Smith, Lisa F. *Girl Walks Out of a Bar: A Memoir* (SelectBooks, 2016)

Smith, Nadia *True to My Roots* (Balboa Press, 2017)

Thomson, Janet *The Placebo Diet: Use Your Mind to Transform Your Body* (True to Our Roots, 2019) (Hay House, 2016)

Tozer, Amber *Sober Stick Figure* (Running Press, 2016)

Trimpey, Jack *Rational Recovery: The New Cure for Substance Addiction* (Pocket Books, 1996)

Vale, Jason *Kick the Drink... Easily!* (Crown House, 2011)
Vale, Jason *7lbs in 7 days: Super Juice Diet* (Harper Thorsons, 2014)
Ware, Bronnie *The Top Five Regrets of the Dying: A Life Transformed by the Dearly Departing* (Hay House, 2019)
Warrington, Ruby *Sober Curious: The Blissful Sleep, Greater Focus, Limitless Presence, and Deep Connection Awaiting Us All on the Other Side of Alcohol* (HarperOne, 2018)
Weller, Rebecca *A Happier Hour* (Mod by Dom, 2016)
Whittaker, Holly Glenn *Quit like a Woman: The Radical Choice to Not Drink in a Culture Obsessed with Alcohol* (Bloomsbury, 2020)
Willoughby, Laura; Tolvi, Jussi; Jaegar, Dru et al. (The Club Soda Community) *How to be a Mindful Drinker: Cut down, stop for a bit, or quit* (DK, 2019)

Audiobooks

Burroughs, Augusten *Lust & Wonder* (St Martin's Griffin, 2017)
Burroughs, Augusten *Dry: A Memoir* (Macmillan Audio, 2003)
Harrold, Glenn and Grace, Janey Lee *Joyful Pregnancy* (Diviniti Publishing, 2007)
Harrold, Glenn and Grace, Janey Lee *Blissful Birth* (Diviniti Publishing, 2007)
Harrold, Glenn and Grace, Janey Lee *Quit the Alcohol Habit* (Diviniti Publishing, 2020)

CONTRIBUTORS

Thank you to our contributors.

I'm immensely grateful for the individuals who contributed to this book, or whose work I have referenced. Thank you for sharing your expertise, it's so appreciated, you've all had a profound effect on me! In no particular order:

Dr Michael Barnish www.revivgloballtd.com
Camille Vidal La Maison Wellness
   www.lamaisonwellness.com/recipes
Jo Wilson & Andy Coley www.beyondnlptraining.com
Peter Donn www.eft-courses.org.uk
Lucy Blenkinsopp www.lucyblenkinsopp.co.uk
Dr Aric Sigman www.aricsigman.com
Janet Thomson www.theplacebodiet.co.uk
Star Khechara www.starkhechara.com and
   www.academyofbeautynutrition.com
Laura Willoughby Club Soda www.joinclubsoda.com
Millie Gooch www.sobergirlsociety.com
William Porter www.alcoholexplained.com
David Hamilton www.drdavidhamilton.com
Rebekah Shaman www.rebekahshaman.com
Jo and Dominic De Rosa www.blissfulinfinity.com/cacao
Nadia Smith www.truetoourroots.co.uk
Hollie Holden www.hollieholden.me
Dr Gemma Newman www.plantpowerdoctor.com
Katie Ruane www.thefamilynaturopath.co.uk

Keilly Natalie Foster www.Fitafcoaching.com
Ciara Jean Roberts www.whollyaligned.com
Beverley Densham www.mindfulnesspilates.com
Caroline Shola Arewa www.energy4lifecoach.com
Heather Dawn Godfrey www.aromantique.co.uk and
    www.InnerTraditions.com
Quantum Sobriety www.quantumsobriety.com
Jolene Park www.grayareadrinkers.com
Glenn Harrold www.glennharrold.com
Sharon Walters www.londonartist1.com
Robyn Spens www.robynspens.com
Stress Management Society www.stress.org.uk
Karla McLaren www.karlamclaren.com
Dr Hannah Short www.drhannahshort.co.uk
Katie Brindle www.hayoumethod.com/
Helena Cavan www.milestonedetox.com and
    www.waterforlife.me
Euan MacLennan www.pukkaherbs.com
James and Vanessa Jacoby www.senserspirits.com
Tam Johnson www.freshinsightcoaching.com
Andy Coley and Jo Wilson www.beyondnlptraining.com

RECOMMENDED RESOURCES

Therapists, coaches, psychologists

(Please note some have contributed to the book, so details can be found under Contributors.)

To find a holistic therapist go to www.fht.org.uk
To find a functional medicine doctor
    www.ifm.org/find-a-practitioner
Family Constellations www.familyconstellationsherts.co.uk
Sleep and nutrition www.robhobson.com
Dr David Snyder www.nlppower.com
Gabor Mate www.drgabormate.com
Tawny Lara www.tawnylara.com
TRE www.traumaprevention.com
Jonathan Haidt www.jonathanhaidt.com
Gabriele Oettingen
    https://as.nyu.edu/content/nyu-as/as/faculty/
    gabriele-oettingen.html

Podcasts

Alcohol Free Life Podcast from The Sober Club
1000 Days Sober
Love Sober
The Rich Roll Podcast
The Bubble Hour

TEDx talks

Janey Lee Grace – Sobriety Rocks – Who Knew!
Jolene Park – Gray Area Drinking
Johann Hari – Everything you think you know about addiction is wrong

Hypnosis audios

www.glennharrold.com

Sober communities

The Sober Club with Janey Lee Grace, where we focus on optimum health and wellbeing underpinned by sobriety, membership includes our online course Get the Buzz without the Booze.
www.thesoberclub.com
This Naked Mind – Annie Grace's community
   www.thisnakedmind.com
Club Soda www.joinclubsoda.co.uk
For younger gals
   Sober Girl Society with Millie Gooch www.sobergirlsociety.com

Buy alcohol free drinks – online drinks retailers

Wise Bartender www.wisebartender.co.uk
Dry Drinker www.drydrinker.com
Booze Free www.boozefree.uk
No and Lo www.drinknolow.com
Club Soda Guide www.clubsodaguide.com

Inspiration/recipes

Camille Vidal La Maison Wellness
www.lamaisonwellness.com/recipes

Alcohol free drinks

Sea Arch www.searachdrinks.com
Jeffrey's Tonics www.jeffreystonics.com

Nonsuch Drinks www.nonsuchdrinks.com
Gin-esque www.oldcoachhousedistillery.com
Sipling Mocktails www.siplingbotanics.com
Wild Life Botanicals www.wildlifebotanicals.com
Noughty Alcohol Free Sparkling wine www.thomsonandscott.com
Binary botanicals www.binarybotanicals.co.uk
Boucha Kombucha www.bouchakombucha.com
Atopia www.atopia.com
Lyres www.lyres.co
Senser Spirits www.senserspirits.com and www.sentiaspirits.com

Pop-up alcohol-free bars

Conscious Bar
See The Sober Club website for individual retailers and recipes

'Dry' bars and restaurants 'embracing' alcohol-free (AF) drinks

Redemption Bar, London
Brewdog AF Bar, London
The Virgin Mary, Dublin
Dishoom, London, Manchester, Edinburgh
The Alchemist, London, Birmingham, Manchester

Sober socialising

Morning Gloryville www.morninggloryville.com
Sober comedy nights www.soberisfun.co.uk

Sober retreats

The Sober Club Selfcare in Sobriety retreats at Champneys
We Love Lucid www.welovelucid.com
Detox retreats www.milestonedetox.com

Sobriety, one-to-one coaching and counselling

Grey Area Drinking, NLP, Health Coaching

Janey Lee Grace

janey@janeyleegrace.com and www.thesoberclub.com
Lee Davy 1000 Days sober www.1000dayssober.com
Rachel Welford www.welfordwellbeing.com

Drug and addiction counselling

Stephanie Chivers www.ichange21.com

Recovery support and information

Club Soda www.joinclubsoda.com
Alcohol Change UK www.alcoholchange.org.uk
Intervention service Forward Together
    www.forward-together.org.uk
Behaviour Change Model
    https://sphweb.bumc.bu.edu/otlt/ph-modules/sb/
    behavioralchangetheories/BehavioralChangeTheories6.html
Rational Recovery www.rational.org

For recovery support meetings contact your local area:

AA www.alcoholics-anonymous.org.uk
Smart Recovery www.smartrecovery.org
Refuge Recovery www.refuserecovery.org

Health and wellbeing resources

Check out www.imperfectlynatural.com for recommendations on
    natural products and services
The lowdown on sustainable cosmetics from Environmental
    Working Group www.ewg.org
Women's Environmental Network www.wen.org.uk
Chuckling Goat www.chucklinggoat.co.uk
HayMax www.haymax.biz
www.1000dayssober.com

Sprouting seeds, beans, lentils *et al*.:
www.buywholefoodsonline.co.uk
Jason Vale www.juicemaster.com

Happy Healthy Sober additional resources

To download resources, guides and up-to-date recommendations go to my website: www.happyhealthysober.com

ACKNOWLEDGEMENTS

Keeping this short… a huge thanks to Caroline and Andrew at McNidder & Grace for believing in this book. Thanks to the incredible support I've had from my long-suffering hubby Simon, who also ditched the booze when he found out how great alcohol-free drinks were! Thanks to my kids Sonny, Buddy, Rocky and Lulu who find my 'obsession' with not drinking highly amusing (but some of that will rub off…right?). I don't think I'd have got this party started without Clare Pooley, and a few other quit lit authors and key players in the Sober World, and of course a massive big-up to all my contributors who have shared their knowledge and expertise. Finally, a huge shout-out must go to my online community The Sober Club, they are an amazing bunch of people, so supportive, non-judgemental and kind… Being sober makes you more kind, its official!

Janey

ABOUT THE AUTHOR

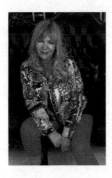

Janey Lee Grace is well known for her appearances on *Steve Wright in the Afternoon – The Big Show* on BBC Radio 2, (9 million listeners) and having a top ten hit record in the 90's with *Cola Boy (Seven Ways To Love)*, touring the world as a backing singer with many stars including George Michael and Wham!, Kim Wilde, and Boy George. She is an Amazon Number One best-selling author of *Imperfectly Natural Woman*. Janey runs the hugely successful health and wellbeing website imperfectlynatural.com and has been voted Number One in 'Who's Who' in Natural Beauty Industry yearbook for three consecutive years. Janey's most recent TV appearances were on *Good Morning Britain* and *Celebrity Antiques Road Trip*, and has made regular contributions on many shows including *The Wright Stuff*, *BBC Breakfast* and Sky TV Entertainment news.

In 2018 Janey decided to ditch the drink and quickly realised that sobriety was the missing piece of the 'holistic health jigsaw'. She hosts Alcohol Free Life Podcast and runs The Sober Club.

www.happyhealthysober.com

www.thesoberclub.com

www.imperfectlynatural.com